Urological Tests in
Clinical Practice

Urological Tests in Clinical Practice

Nagaraja P. Rao, Shalom J. Srirangam and Glenn M. Preminger

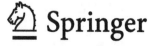 Springer

N. Rao, ChM., FRCS
Consultant Urological Surgeon
Director of Stone Management Unit
Department of Urology
South Manchester University Hospitals NHS Trust
Wythenshawe Hospital
Manchester, UK

S. Srirangam, MD, MRCS
Specialist Registrar in Urology
Department of Urology
South Manchester University Hospitals NHS Trust
Wythenshawe Hospital
Manchester, UK

G. Preminger, MD
Professor of Urologic Surgery
Director, Duke Comprehensive Kidney Stone Center
Duke University Medical Center
Division of Urologic Surgery
Durham, NC, USA

British Library Cataloguing in Publication Data
A catalogue record for this book is available from the British Library

Library of Congress Control Number: 2006922752

ISBN-10: 1-84628-390-6   e-ISBN 1-84628-422-8   Printed on acid-free paper
ISBN-13: 978-1-84628-390-1

9 8 7 6 5 4 3 2 1

Springer Science+Business Media, LLC
springer.com

Preface

As this book was going to press, the Editor-in-Chief of the British Journal of Urology International introduced an interesting and timely phrase "finger tip urology". He has rightly pointed out that medical knowledge base is expanding so rapidly that no urologist can keep pace. The implication is that there is a desperate need for an easy reference source in many areas of urology. We think that this book is "spot on"!

Urological diagnosis is rarely possible without tests. And there are several tests to request. What investigation to order in which patient is always in the mind of those who care for urological patients. We hope that this book helps to resolve some of that dilemma.

The book is in two parts. Part one details the tests urologists today need to do, ranging from simple dipstix testing of urine to MR spectroscopy. No test is of value if one does not know when to apply it. Part two therefore outlines common urological conditions and the tests that need to be performed to reach a diagnosis. There is also a wealth of other information too; to give an example, TNM classification of tumors.

We hope that you as a busy resident in urology, newly appointed urologist, specialist urological nurse or other health professional allied to urology, will find this "finger tip information" of value in the management of common urological problems.

This book obviously contains a lot of information, and though quite substantial, is succinct and may therefore suffer from the usual disadvantage of over simplicity. But that is the whole purpose—providing a quick reference. We hope that you find this handy and useful in your practice.

Best wishes

N.Rao
S.Srirangam
G.Preminger

Contents

Part II: Urological Conditions Requiring Investigations

Part I
Urological Investigations

Chapter 1
Urine Tests

(a) URINALYSIS

Urinalysis is a requisite examination in the assessment of all urological patients and comprises—

A. Physical examination of urine
B. Dipstick analysis
C. Microscopic analysis of urine

Appropriate specimen collection and transport is vital for accurate and clinically valid results.

Specimen collection and transport
Midstream specimen of urine (MSU)
The typically acidic and concentrated early morning urine (EMU) samples are more likely to detect a urinary tract infection (UTI), since red blood cells (RBC), white blood cells (WBC), and casts are best preserved in such a medium. In addition, overnight bacterial proliferation will also increase the yield from EMU samples.

- Males should retract the foreskin, clean the glans penis, and void with the foreskin retracted and collect a mid-stream sample without stopping urine flow
- Females are required to clean the vulva and separate the labia prior to specimen collection

Suprapubic aspiration of urine
- Gold standard technique for the diagnosis of a UTI
- May be required in patients with an equivocal result from an MSU
- Commonly employed in the pediatric population
- Best achieved by a sterile suprapubic puncture (with a spinal needle) under ultrasound guidance

Urine via intermittent catheterization

- Requires passage of a lo-fric® catheter to obtain a urine sample
- Discard initial urine and collect subsequent urine
- Even a sterile intermittent catheterization carries up to a 2% risk of introducing a new UTI

Fractionated urine samples

In males, although MSUs are adequate, in certain clinical conditions it might be appropriate to take different aliquots of urine to aid localization of the UTI (e.g., diagnosis of prostatitis).

- Voided bladder 1 (VB1)—first 5–10 mL of voided urine and represents urethral flora
- Voided bladder 2 (VB2)—mid-stream urine and best correlates with bladder urine
- Voided bladder 3 (VB3)—initial 2–3 mL of urine, containing expressed prostatic secretions (EPS), collected following prostate massage

In patients with a suspected sexually transmitted infection (STI), urethritis, or urethral discharge, a VB1 and VB3 specimen are sent separately for culture.

- A bacterial count greater than 10 times in VB3 compared to VB1 or 2 is diagnostic of prostatitis
- A leucocyte count >10 per high-power field in VB3 compared to VB1 or 2 is diagnostic of prostatitis
- An EPS or VB3 pH of >8 is suggestive of prostatitis
- A higher bacterial count in VB1 compared to VB3 is diagnostic of urethritis

Urine from indwelling catheters

Interpretation of urinalysis from patients on long-term indwelling catheterization is problematic for a variety of reasons, and unnecessary treatment may result in the emergence of antibiotic –resistant organisms.

- Bladder colonization is inevitable and can occur within 4 days of catheter placement
- A positive bacterial growth does not necessarily suggest a significant UTI
- Antibiotic therapy is unlikely to eradicate the targeted pathogen while the patient remains catheterized
- Colonizing flora may change over time

In such patients, a urine sample should only be sent if a UTI is suspected in a systemically unwell patient. Urine must be taken from the collection port and not from the catheter bag.

Urine from ileal conduits
Skin organism contamination is inevitable in patients with urinary diversions and therefore urostomy bag urine is not suitable. If clinically indicated, urine collection should be via a catheter introduced as far into the conduit as it will go.

Urine collection in children
• UTIs are common in children
• Urine collection can be difficult
• Toilet-trained children can provide an MSU
• Urine from children not toilet trained can be obtained by a "clean voided" bag sample, suprapubic aspiration, or transurethral catheterization

The relative merits and drawbacks are discussed in Table 1.1.

Urine transport
• Specimen must reach laboratory within 2 hours
• Delay can result in either over-proliferation or death of organisms
• Alternatively, store at a temperature of 4°C if a delay is encountered and analyze as soon as possible
• Beware that refrigeration can result in a decreased number of urinary leucocytes

A. Physical examination of urine
Color: The endogenously produced pigment, urochrome, gives urine its characteristic yellow-brown color. Since urochrome is excreted at a uniform rate (i.e., the same amount per hour), the color of urine varies primarily with urine output, which in turn is predominantly affected by the patient's hydration status. In addition, a variety of other compounds related to food, medication, and infection can alter the color of urine. Patients commonly complain of altered urine color and it is important to be aware of common urine color-altering factors, as listed in Table 1.2.

Turbidity: Cloudy urine is commonly caused by—
• Phosphaturia—will typically occur after consumption of a large meal or quantity of milk in susceptible patients.

TABLE 1.1. Comparision of urine collection techniques in children

	Clean voided bag samples	Suprapubic aspiration	Urethral catheterization
Technique	Clean perineum and external genitalia. Apply bag. Remove promptly and perform urinalysis after micturition	Insert a 1.5-inch, 22-gauge needle, 1–2 cm above symphysis pubis under ultrasound guidance; aspirate 5 mL of urine	Insert a 5 or 6F urethral catheter into bladder using lidocaine lubricant jelly; discard first few drops of urine
Advantages	Non-invasive	Safe High sensitivity (>95%) Quick	Safe Successful in virtually 100% of cases
Disadvantages	Contamination—high false positive (63%) Positive culture may not be sufficient to commence antibiotic therapy	Hematuria, intestinal or viscus perforation (risk very small) Success rate variable—46–96% Can only be used in children <2 years age	Invasive Urethral trauma/hematuria False positives (80%) Takes longer than suprapubic aspiration Cannot be used in older children
Clinical comments	Positive results usually require validation by using an invasive technique	Gold standard	Correlates reasonably well with suprapubic aspiration

TABLE 1.2. Factors affecting urine color

Color	Causes
Red	Hematuria
	Hemoglobinuria
	Myoglobinuria
	Beet-root
	Blackberries
	Rifampicin
	Heavy metal poisoning (mercury, lead)
Yellow	Riboflavin
	Phenacetin
Orange	Concentrated urine (dehydration)
	Phenazopyridine
	Sulfasalazine
Blue or green	Biliverdin
	Dyes (methylene blue, indigo carmine)
	Cimetidine
	Promethazine
Brown	Hemorrhage
	Laxatives (e.g., senna)
	Urobilinogen
	Porphyria
	Rhubarb
	Aloe
	Anti-malarials (e.g., chloroquine)
	Antibiotics (e.g., nitrofurantoin, metronidazole)
	Methyldopa

Diagnosis is completed by either acidifying the alkaline urine to dissolve the excess phosphate crystals (urine turns clear) or by visualizing the precipitated phosphate crystals under microscopy
- UTI—pungent-smelling, cloudy urine is likely to be secondary to pyuria associated with an infective process
- Rare causes of turbid urine include chyluria (lymph fluid in urine), hyperoxaluria, and lipiduria

B. Urine dipstick analysis
Dipstick testing is useful in assessing patients with—

- Renal disease
- Urological disorders
- Metabolic disease not related to the kidneys

TABLE 1.3. Reference range for urine dipstick parameters

	Adult	Child
Color	Light straw to dark amber	Light straw to dark yellow
Turbidity	Clear	Clear
Odour	Aromatic	Aromatic
Specific gravity	1.005–1.040	1.005–1.030 (1.005–1.020 in newborns)
pH	4.5–8.0	4.5–8.0
Blood	Negative	Negative
Protein	Negative	Negative
Glucose	Negative	Negative
Ketones	Negative	Negative

Urine dipsticks use reagent strips, where a chemical reaction with an active compound results in color changes that provide important information on (1) urinary specific gravity, (2) pH, (3) blood, (4) protein, (5) glucose, (6) ketones, (7) WBC, (8) nitrites, and (9) bilirubin and urobilinogen. Normal findings are highlighted in Table 1.3.

Specific gravity (SG)
- Measure of total solute concentration
- Usually varies between 1.001 and 1.040
- SG of >1.020 is concentrated
- SG of <1.008 is considered dilute

The state of hydration and renal insufficiency are the two main determinants of urine SG.

- SG decreases with age as the renal concentrating ability diminishes
- Over-hydration, diuretic therapy, diabetes insipidus, and renal failure will all result in a decreased urine SG
- In renal failure (acute or chronic) the kidneys lose the ability to concentrate urine and the SG remains fixed at 1.010

pH
- Urinary pH ranges from 4.5 to 8
- pH of <5.5 is considered acidic
- pH of >6.5 regarded alkaline
- Urinary pH changes rapidly when in contact with air; therefore, prompt testing is essential

As a general rule, urinary pH reflects serum pH, but there is an important exception.

- In renal tubular acidosis (RTA), the urine will often remain alkaline in spite of the presence of acidic urine, due to urinary bicarbonate loss
- In severe type II RTA (proximal) the urine may occasionally become acidic, but will always remain alkaline even with severe type I RTA (distal)

Additionally, alkaline urine (pH over 7.5) suggests infection by a urea-splitting organism such as *Proteus*. Vegetarians commonly have alkaline urine due to low acid ingestion. Uric acid and cystine stones form in acidic urine (pH less than 5.5).

Blood
- Detection of blood is due to peroxidase-like activity of hemoglobin, which catalyzes the oxidation of a chromogen indicator, causing a color change in direct proportion to the amount of blood in urine
- Hematuria, hemoglobinuria, and myoglobinuria will all result in positive dipstick for blood
- Dipstick detection of hematuria (defined at >3 RBC/high-power field) has a sensitivity of over 90%
- There is also a higher false-positive rate

Common causes of false-positive results include—

(i)   Urine contamination with menstrual blood
(ii) Dehydration
(iii) Exercise
(iv) Oxidizing agents
(v)   Bacterial peroxidase

False-negative results may occur with poorly mixed urine or with patients on high doses of vit C. Microscopic evaluation is mandatory in any patients with positive dipstick test for hematuria.

Protein
- Proteinuria in adults is defined as the excretion of >150 mg of protein per day (normal protein excretion rate is 80–150 mg)
- Dipstick analysis will detect concentrations as low as 10 mg/dL

The protein concentration of urine alters the urine pH and this results in a change in the color of the pH-sensitive dye on the dipstick. Albumin, the primary urinary protein, causes the dipstick to turn green; the darker the green, the greater the urinary protein concentration.

Causes of false negatives include—

• Alkaline urine
• Dilute urine
• Urine in which albumin is not the primary protein

The detection of proteinuria on a dipstick is a measure of protein concentration and not protein excretion; therefore, measurement of 24-hour urinary protein excretion and protein electrophoresis is mandatory to rule out underlying renal disease.

Proteinuria can be classified by timing into—

1. Transient: common; occurs in children; also in patients with sepsis, cardiac failure and following exercise; spontaneous resolution
2. Intermittent: occurs in young men in the upright position due to increased renal vein pressure; not pathological
3. Persistent: pathological and requires further evaluation with 24-hour urine collection for protein excretion

(Proteinuria is further discussed in the section on 24-hour urine collection. Section 1f–page 28)

Glucose
Detection occurring due to a double oxidative reaction of the glucose with glucose oxidase on the dipstick is specific for glucose and does not occur with any other sugars. Patients with a positive glucose dipstick should be investigated for diabetes mellitus.

• Glucosuria should not be present in the normal healthy adult
• A positive dipstick suggests that the renal tubular reabsorption threshold has been exceeded. This corresponds to a serum glucose level of about 18 mg/L
• Nevertheless, the degree of glucosuria correlates poorly with hyperglycemia

Ketones
• Ketones (acetoacetic acid and acetone) are detected by the nitroprusside test

- Not usually present in urine from healthy adults
- Frequently associated with catabolic situations (with increased breakdown of body fat) such as diabetic ketoacidosis, starvation, and pregnancy

WBC

Pyuria is detected either by dipstick or microscopy. Leucocyte esterase, a leucocyte-specific isoenzyme, is the basis for dipstick testing. Common causes include—

- UTI
- Tumors
- Stones
- Glomerulonephritis
- Foreign bodies
- Fungal infection
- Tuberculosis
- Certain drugs (e.g., cyclophosphamide)

False-positive tests occur due to contamination. False-negative results are usually due to—

- Inadequate contact of dipstick with urine
- Increased urinary specific gravity
- Glycosuria
- Presence of urobilinogen
- Ascorbic acid in urine

Therefore leucocyte esterase in isolation is insufficient to diagnose a UTI, but in conjunction with positive urinary nitrites is strongly suggestive of infection. Its use should be confined to screening urine in the asymptomatic patient in the primary care setting.

Nitrites

- Common urinary gram-negative bacteria can convert nitrates to nitrites
- A positive nitrite dipstick has a high specificity for detecting bacteriuria (>90%) but its sensitivity is variable (40–85%). Accuracy is also diminished in subclinical bacteriuria (<10^5 organism/mL)
- Contamination can result in a false-positive result
- In the hospital setting, urine dipstick for leucocyte esterase and nitrites is not an adequate replacement for urine microscopy and culture in the detection of urinary tract infection

Bilirubin and urobilinogen
- Normal adult urine should contain very little urobilinogen and no bilirubin
- Patients with liver disease and biliary obstruction will have elevated levels of conjugated bilirubin which is water-soluble and will be detectable on dipstick
- Urinary bilirubin is pathological and warrants hepatobiliary investigations
- Urobilinogen is the end product of conjugated bilirubin metabolism, but is also increasingly detectable in urine in patients with hemolysis, hepatocellular disease, and gastrointestinal hemorrhage

C. Urine microscopy
Urine microscopy is useful, reliable, and cheap. Indications include—

- Suspected UTI
- Suspected acute glomerulonephritis
- Unexplained acute or chronic renal failure
- Hematuria
- Suspected urinary tract malignancy

Technique
- Obtain a clean catch, first morning (preferably) urine sample MSU
- About 10–15 mL is centrifuged at 3,000 rpm for 5 minutes, with the supernatant subsequently discarded
- 0.01–0.02 mL of the residual sediment is placed directly on the microscope slide and covered with a coverslip
- Microscopy should include examination at both low power (×100 magnification) and high power (×400 magnification). Low-power magnification is adequate for the identification of most cells, macrophages, and parasites, but high-power is required to discriminate between circular and dysmorphic RBC, and to identify crystals, bacteria, and yeast
- Careful inspection is performed for (1) cells, (2) casts, (3) crystals, (4) bacteria, (5) yeast, and (6) parasites

It is prudent to remember that the volume of urine visualized in one HPF represents 1/30,000 mL and false negatives, due to this volume constraint, are therefore inevitable.

I. Cells

RBC
Urine containing less than 3 RBC per HPF is considered normal. Microscopy is superior to urine dipstick in detection of hematuria (greater than 3 erythrocytes/HPF). Although both tests have a similar sensitivity, the specificity of dipstick analysis is lower (about 70%). Microscopy can also distinguish between hemoglobinuria (large number of erythrocytes seen) and myoglobinuria (erythrocytes absent).

Additional features can assist in localizing the origin of hematuria in glomerular and non-glomerular causes (see Table 1.4).

WBC
Pyuria is best diagnosed by microscopic examination of centrifuged urine sediment. Normal urine may contain up to 2 WBC per HPF in men, and up to 5 WBC per HPF in women. Significant pyuria requires >10 WBC per HPF.

- Fresh leucocytes (larger and rounder) are more suggestive of pathology, while old leucocytes (small and wrinkled) are usually seen in urine contaminated with vaginal secretions
- Large numbers of WBCs per HPF is highly specific for UTIs (especially if associated with hematuria), but various factors can affect the numbers of WBCs detected, including the intensity of the inflammatory response; hydration status of the patient; urine collection technique; and centrifugation and sampling technique
- Other causes of significant pyuria include almost any non-infective urinary tract pathology and results must be interpreted appropriately. Persistent abacterial pyuria should instigate investigations to exclude—
  - Urinary stones
  - Tumors
  - Urinary tuberculosis
  - Glomerulonephritis

The absence of pyuria, in conjunction with either a negative bacterial culture or with a growth of mixed organisms, is likely to be secondary to contamination. Moreover, even with isolation of a single urinary pathogen, the absence of pyuria would suggest a contamination/sampling error in over 85% of patients.

TABLE 1.4. Origin of hematuria in glomerular and non-glomerular causes

	Glomerular	Non-glomerular	
		Renal	Urological
Erythrocyte morphology	Typically dysmorphic (rarely round) Minimal hemoglobin Irregular cytoplasm distribution	Circular/normal morphology	Circular/normal morphology
Associated proteinuria	Significant proteinuria (2+ to 3+ on dipstick, 100–200 mg/dL)	Usually significant proteinuria	Usually absent
Casts	Usually contains red blood cell casts	Casts absent	Casts absent
Causes	Glomerulonephritis (GN) IgA nephropathy (Berger's disease) Mesangioproliferative GN Focal segmental proliferate GN Familial GN (Alport's syndrome) Membranous GN	Polycystic kidney disease Medullary sponge kidney Papillary necrosis Coagulopathy Renal tumors Exercise-induced Renal artery embolism/thrombosis Renal vein thrombosis	Urological tumors Stones UTI
Action	Serum creatinine 24-hour urine for protein excretion Referral to nephrologist Renal biopsy?	Rule out urological cause Treat underlying condition?	Urine cytology Cystoscopy Renal tract imaging

Epithelial cells

Microscopy may also reveal squamous, transitional, and renal tubular cells.

- Squamous cells originate from the vagina, urethra, or trigone and typically appear large with irregular cytoplasm and a small, central nucleus
- Transitional cells are smaller with prominent cytoplasm staining, and have a large nucleus. The features of malignant transitional cells are discussed later in the chapter on urine cytology
- Renal tubular cells are larger and uncommon but, if present, suggest a glomerular pathology

2. Casts

The Tamm–Horsfall mucoprotein, excreted by the renal tubular epithelial cells, forms the basic medium for all renal casts by entrapping any cells (e.g., RBC, WBC, and sloughed renal tubular cells) within the tubular lumen. Hyaline casts, containing only mucoproteins, are excreted normally and therefore are not considered pathological. Conditions that increase hyaline cast excretion include pyelonephritis, chronic renal failure, and physical exercise.

Careful microscopic inspection of cast contents will disclose a number of underlying conditions (see Table 1.5).

3. Crystals

A number of distinct crystals can be identified in the urine of normal patients, but are more frequently seen in the urine of patients with stone disease. Crystal precipitation is dependant on urine pH.

TABLE 1.5. Urinary casts

Casts	Clinical Significance
Hyaline	Present in normal urine ($\uparrow$ in dehydration and proteinuria)
Red blood cells	Glomerular bleeding due to glomerulonephritis
White blood cells	Seen in acute pyelonephritis and acute glomerulonephritis
Cellular	Nonspecific renal damage resulting in sloughing of renal tubular cells
Fatty	Commonly seen in nephritic syndrome, lipiduria and hypothyroidism

- Alkaline urine → calcium phosphate, calcium triphosphate (struvite) crystals
- Acidic urine → calcium oxalate, uric acid and cystine stones

Crystals are discussed in more detail in the chapter on urine analysis for stones.

4. Bacteria

Although the results of urine culture are far more important than the results of microscopy, in the diagnosis of a UTI, an effort should be made to detect bacteria on urine microscopy, as normal urine is sterile and should contain no bacteria.

Nevertheless, contamination, either from poor sampling technique or vaginal/peri-urethral flora in a female, can often result in positive identification in urine. In males, detection of any bacteria should prompt further evaluation with a urine specimen. In females, a count of 5 bacteria/HPF reflects a colony count of about 100,000 organisms/mL and is diagnostic of a UTI.

The morphology of any observed bacteria can provide useful clues. The most common uropathogens are aerobic gram-negative rods and these have a characteristic bacillary shape. *Staphylococci* are seen in clumps, whereas *streptococci* typically form beaded chains. The presence of filamentous *lactobacilli* is suggestive of vaginal floral contamination.

5. Yeast

Candida albicans is the most common yeast cell found in urine, especially in patients with diabetes mellitus or long-term in-dwelling urinary catheters. Contamination can occur from a vaginal source. The characteristic appearance of *Candida* with budding and hyphae formation distinguishes it from other microorganisms.

6. Parasites

Patients with schistosomiasis (*S. hematobium*) usually originate from, or have travelled to North Africa or the Middle East, and inspection of their urine during the early/middle stage may reveal the characteristic parasitic ovum with its terminal spike. Examination of a terminal specimen of urine yields best results.

Trichomonas vaginalis are large flagellated organisms which can be easily seen in patients with urethritis.

Urine culture
- Diagnosis of a UTI requires bacterial growth in urine culture
- Urine should be cultured immediately or refrigerated at 4°C and analyzed within 24 hours

Although various techniques of urine culture and bacterial count estimation have been described, the standard surface plating and dip-slide methods are the most widely used.

Technique
1. **Standard surface plating**: a standard loop is dipped in urine (0.1 mL) and inoculated onto an agar plate. One half of the agar plate is blood agar (grows any bacteria), while the other is a more selective medium, such as MacConkey or eosin-ethylene blue, which grows gram-negative bacteria. Each bacterial rod or cocci cluster will form a colony after overnight incubation, which can be counted, identified, and multiplied by 10 to report the number of colony-forming units (cfu) per mL of urine. This technique is reasonably accurate and is widely recommended.

2. **Dip-slide method**: is simpler, less expensive, and less accurate than standard surface plating. A commercially available, double-sided, agar coated slide is dipped in urine, incubated overnight in its sterile container and the approximate bacterial count estimated by reading off a supplied picture chart. This semiquantitative method is useful for general practices or remote medical centers.

Interpretation
Though it is well recognized that significant bacteriuria represents a count of greater than 10^5 cfu/mL, this is perhaps an oversimplification

- Urine is a good culture medium (with a bacterial doubling time of 30–45 minutes) and, if allowed to incubate long enough, most bacteria will reach a count level of 10^5 cfu/mL
- Therefore "significant bacteriuria" only applies if the sample has been collected, transported, and cultured appropriately
- Nevertheless, 70–80% of women with a UTI will have 10^5 cfu/mL
- The majority of women with counts of <10^2 cfu/mL do not have a UTI and bacterial growth is due to contamination or delay in specimen transport

- A third of women with acute cystitis symptoms have a count of between 10^2 and 10^4 cfu/mL. In these patients, the commonly isolated pathogens include *E. coli*, *Proteus*, and *S. saprophyticus*. Therefore, in the symptomatic female, the appropriate threshold for defining "significant bacteriuria" is 10^2 cfu/mL of a known pathogen. A likely explanation for this phenomenon may be that frequent voids in symptomatic patients result in a decreased colony count
- Counts of $>10^5$ cfu/mL are due to contamination in up to 20% of patients (either from the vagina/perineum in infection-susceptible women or the foreskin in uncircumcised men)
- Contamination in men is uncommon; therefore, counts of 10^2 cfu/mL in a well-collected urine sample should be considered significant
- Identification of any bacteria in urine obtained by sterile suprapubic aspiration is clinically significant

Significant bacteriuria in adults in clinical practice can therefore be summarized as follows:

Females
- MSU showing $>10^3$ cfu/mL with acute uncomplicated cystitis
- MSU showing $>10^4$ cfu/mL with acute uncomplicated pyelonephritis
- MSU showing $>10^5$ cfu/mL with a complicated UTI

Males
- MSU showing $>10^4$ cfu/mL with a complicated UTI

Features that are indicative of a true UTI include—

1. Symptomatic patient
2. Single organism isolated
3. Repeat culture identifies same uropathogen
4. Pyuria (>10 WBC/HPF)
5. Significant bacteriuria (≥ 10 cfu/mL suprapubic aspiration or $>10^4$ cfu/mL from MSU)

Be aware that patients with a high fluid intake, urinary frequency, and/or on antibiotics may have a decreased bacterial count.

Features which decrease the likelihood of a UTI include—

1. No urinary symptoms
2. Mixed bacterial growth
3. Count $<10^4$ cfu/mL
4. No pyuria
5. Epithelial cells or lactobacilli on microscopy suggests vaginal contamination

---

(b) FLOW CYTOMETRY (DNA PLOIDY)

Introduction

Tumors are characterized by a higher percentage of proliferating cells, and therefore the presence of increased mitotic figures correlates with tumor aggressiveness in transitional cell carcinoma (TCC) of the urinary tract. Flow cytometry (FCM) can measure the DNA content of cells, and therefore objectively quantitate the aneuploid cell population and the proliferative activity (proportion of cells in S phase of the cell cycle) within a tumor.

Indications

Due to the fact that FCM has not demonstrated clinical superiority over urine cytology, its use remains sporadic. Potential indications include—

* As a screening tool, in combination with urine cytology, for the high-risk patient group
* As a prognostic indicator of muscle invasiveness
* As a predictor of recurrence, in combination with morphonuclear scoring
* To assess efficacy of intravesical therapy for TCC of the bladder

Specimen collection and analysis

* A large number of cells are required for pertinent analysis, and less than 50% of voided specimens have adequate cellularity for FCM
* Up to one-third have uninterpretable histograms due to cell degeneration in unfixed specimen
* Although FCM is best performed on bladder irrigation specimens, fresh, frozen or paraffin-embedded tumor tissues can also be used

To prevent cell degeneration, bladder irrigation samples must either be analyzed immediately, refrigerated and tested within 24 hours, or frozen for subsequent use.

Interpretation
- The majority of normal urothelial cells as well as grade I TCC are DNA diploid
- Most grade III are DNA aneuploid
- Suspect CIS if bladder irrigation specimen is DNA aneuploid and bladder biopsy DNA diploid

The majority of patients (97%) with cytological diagnosis of cancer have abnormal DNA ploidy, but only 5% of patients with normal cytology have abnormal DNA ploidy (see Table 1.6)

Prognosis: Grade II TCC are a heterogeneous group with equal numbers of DNA diploid and aneuploid cases. DNA ploidy adds more prognostic information in this group than the grade itself. In the superficial grade II TCC, the 5-year recurrence-free rates are 75% for DNA diploid compared to 25% for DNA aneuploid. In general, the trend with regards to prognosis is diploid > tetraploid > triploid to tetraploid.

Progression: In superficial TCC (grade I/II), progression to muscle invasion, in a tumor containing DNA diploid, DNA tetraploid, and DNA aneuploid cell populations, occurred in 2%, 10% and 50% of patients respectively. Nearly all grade III patients are aneuploid and FCM is not of value in their prognosis.

Survival: In CIS, the 5-year progression-free survival in patients with one and multiple DNA aneuploid populations is 67% and 20%, respectively. The mean survival time for DNA diploid T3a or less is 91 months versus 26 months for DNA aneuploid T3b or T4. Patients with low S-phase fractions (<11%) also have a longer recurrence-free survival than those with higher values.

Recurrence: The presence of a clear non-tetraploid DNA histogram is diagnostic of recurrent TCC. In patients with atypical cytological findings, 20% with abnormal DNA ploidy have a recurrence compared to only 5% with normal DNA ploidy. Combining FCM with cytology has a 95% sensitivity in detecting recurrent TCC in the bladder, with no loss of specificity. In

TABLE 1.6. DNA ploidy

DNA Status	Cytology Negative (%)
DNA diploid	98
DNA tetraploid	69
DNA aneuploid	8

addition, combining FCM with the morphonuclear score (an image analysis-based nuclear grading system) recurrence versus non-recurrence is predicted in 91% of low-grade disease.

Treatment monitoring: Patients treated with radiotherapy for muscle-invasive TCC have a clinical response in 100%, 54%, and 30% of cases for tumor that are DNA diploid, aneuploid, and multiploid, respectively. About 70% of patients with an S-phase fraction <11% survive 10 years in contrast to only 30% of patients with a fraction value of >11%. After radiotherapy, a DNA tetraploid population can be expected up to 2 years post-therapy and should not be interpreted as treatment failure.

The presence of DNA diploid cells in patients undergoing intravesical chemotherapy indicates a good response, whereas an aneuploid DNA histogram indicates treatment failure.

Drawbacks
- Invasive procedure (catheterization for specimen collection)
- Large number of cells required
- Only significant DNA chromosomal abnormalities lead to changes in the DNA ploidy detectable by FCM and minor chromosomal abnormalities are missed
- Not all TCC is associated with an abnormal DNA content
- FCM equipment not available in all units

- FCM measures cell DNA content (the degree of aneuploidy)
- Most grade III are DNA aneuploid
- 97% of patients with TCC and abnormal cytology have abnormal DNA ploidy
- Abnormal DNA ploidy is associated with poor prognosis (higher recurrence and progression, poorer response to treatment)
- General prognostic trend is diploid > tetraploid > triploid to tetraploid

---

(c) CYTOLOGY

Introduction
Urothelial cells are constantly being exfoliated into urine in both normal patients and those with transitional cell carcinoma (TCC)

of the urinary tract. These cells can be identified, fixed, and analyzed in order to determine cell morphology, thereby providing a convenient, non-invasive technique for the observation of high-risk patients. As a gold standard, voided urine cytology (VUC) is unquestionably inadequate and is plagued with problems of poor sensitivity. Nevertheless, while emerging novel urinary markers for the detection of TCC still remain largely unproven, VUC will have widespread use.

Indications
- Surveillance or screening for TCC or CIS in the urinary tract
- Frank hematuria in any patient >40 years of age
- Irritative lower urinary tract symptom in any patient >40 years of age (to detect CIS)

Specimen collection and analysis
One variable affecting the sensitivity of urine cytology is the type of specimen. Voided urine is easy to obtain, but generally hypocellular and degenerated. Contamination by skin and vaginal contents may also occur in females. The sensitivity is augmented when three specimens are obtained on separate days. For one, two, and three voided specimens, sensitivities of 41%, 41%, and 60% have been reported respectively.

- *Voided urine*: an early-morning sample is not suitable and the second morning provides the best specimen. Collect 50 mL in a universal container and send to the lab immediately
- *Catheterized urine samples and bladder washouts*: these have a higher cellularity and less contamination, but require an invasive procedure that may introduce instrument artefact. In addition, urine from patients with an indwelling catheter is unsuitable for analysis, as denuded normal epithelial cells may be interpreted as low-grade TCC. Saline bladder washouts are three times as accurate (80% for CIS) as voided urine since the mechanical action of barbotage enhances tumor cell shedding and better preserves for examination
- *Ureteric urine sampling*: the ureter is catheterized up to a point just below the level of suspected lesion. Urine from the other ureter is sent for control. False-negative rates are high (22% to 35%), but saline washes will improve overall sensitivity. Brush biopsy performed via a retrograde catheter improves yield, with a reported sensitivity of 91%, a specificity of 88%, and an

accuracy of 89%. Complications include ureteric bleeding and perforation

Analysis
- Urine must be sent for analysis as soon as possible after collection
- Following centrifuge, the cell pellet obtained is divided between two slides
- One is stained with Papanicolaou stain and the other with hematoxylin and eosin
- Microscopic analysis is performed

Interpretation
Primary goals of VUC are to—

- Recognize early flat lesions such as CIS before they invade
- Detect the 10% of superficial lesions destined to invade

Characteristically, TCC cells may appear singly or in small clusters, have large hyperchromatic nuclei with irregular, coarsely textured chromatin. Malignant cells identified in cytological specimens may be classified as—

- Low grade—correlate with histological grade I lesions and some grade II lesions
- High grade—correlate with some grade II lesions, all grade III lesions, and also with CIS

In patients who are observed for bladder TCC, the overall sensitivity of positive urine cytology is approximately 40–60%, but the sensitivity increases to about 90% for high grade disease and CIS.

A positive cytological diagnosis is highly predictive of TCC, even in the presence of normal cystoscopy. Malignant cells may appear in the urine long before cystoscopically detectable lesions emerge, leading to a seemingly inflated rate of false-positive results. The overall reported false-negative rate is 65%, but may be as high as 96% in low-grade tumors.

High-grade TCC and CIS
- VUC has excellent performance statistics in patients with high-grade lesion, and as such justifies its use as a screening and surveillance device
- Sensitivity is at least 90%

- Specificity reaches 98–100%
- Cells shed from CIS have a similar cytomorphology as high-grade invasive lesions

Low-grade TCC

- Due to the fact that cells of low-grade well-differentiated tumors closely resemble normal urothelial cells, cytologists often opt for terminology such as "atypical cells present" or "cannot rule out low-grade lesion"
- Varying sensitivities of 0–100%
- Specificities ranging from 6–100%
- Efforts continue to be focused on the development of ancillary techniques to improve the sensitivity of VUC in low-grade disease

Positive cytology with no discernible lesion in the bladder or urethra should prompt further investigation of the upper urinary tract. The overall sensitivity of cytology can be improved with multiple voided specimens or bladder washings. Combining VUC with flow cytometry to detect malignant cells with abnormal DNA can also increase yield.

Disadvantages

- Overall high false-negative rate (80% for low-grade TCC, up to 20% for high-grade)
- Subjectivity: greatest determinant of sensitivity of VUC is the level of cytopathologist expertise
- Artifacts may occur in the presence of urolithiasis, inflammation, indwelling catheter, recent instrumentation, intravesical therapy, bowel substitution for bladder, and following chemo- or radiotherapy. Cellular changes may persist for up to a year following treatment
- Contamination with vaginal, cervical, or endometrial cells in women may result in misinterpretation

---

- Indicated in patients >40 years of age with frank hematuria and/or irritative LUTS or as part of TCC surveillance
- Excellent specificity (>98%) and sensitivity (>90%) for high-grade disease and CIS
- Positive VUC is highly predictive of TCC (even if urinary tract endoscopy normal)
- Significant drawbacks (subjectivity and artefacts)

(d) GLOMERULAR FILTRATION RATE

Introduction

Normal values —125–130 mL/min/1.73 m²
               —values vary with age and gender
               —GFR declines by approx. 10 mL/min/1.73 m² per
                 decade after the 4th decade of life
               —GFR <10 mL/min/1.73 m² requires consideration
                 for dialysis or renal transplant

The glomerular filtration rate (GFR)—

1. Remains the most accurate index of renal function
2. Is reduced before the onset of kidney disease
3. When decreased, correlates with the pathological severity of the disease

Indications

- Detection or monitoring of patients with existing renal failure, or at risk of developing renal failure
- Establish renal function prior to administration of potentially nephrotoxic therapy (e.g., chemotherapy)

The global GFR is dependent on the total number of functioning nephron units, such that—

$$GFR = N \ (total \ number \ of \ nephrons) \times GFR \ of \ a \ single \ nephron$$

Therefore, a decrease in the number of nephrons, as well as a reduction in the GFR of a single nephron due to physiological or pharmacological alterations will result in a declining total GFR. Commonly encountered factors affecting GFR are listed below:

- Renal disease (reduced nephron numbers)
- Pregnancy
- Hypovolemia resulting in reduced renal perfusion
- Non-steroidal anti-inflammatory drugs
- Acute protein load/chronic high protein intake
- Hyperglycemia (diabetes)
- High or low blood pressures
- Antihypertensive drugs
- Antibiotic therapy (e.g., aminoglycosides)

GFR is estimated from the urinary clearance of an ideal filtration marker, which is not protein bound in the serum, freely filtered by the kidney, and not reabsorbed or secreted by the nephron. Inulin is the gold standard for GFR measurement, but since its administration and measurement is cumbersome, it remains primarily confined to the research laboratory.

A variety of formulae have been devised to predict the GFR. The most popular are the Cockcroft and Gault equation and the Modification of Diet in Renal Disease (MDRD) equation.

(Cockcroft and Gault)

In males,

$$GFR = \frac{[140 - age\ (y)] \times weight\ (kg) \times 1.23}{serum\ creatinine\ (\mu mol/L)}$$

In females,

$$GFR = \frac{[140 - age\ (y)] \times weight\ (kg) \times 1.04}{serum\ creatinine\ (\mu mol/L)}$$

(Abbreviated MDRD)

GFR = 183 × (serum creatinine) − 1.154 × (age) − 0.203 × (0.742 if female) (×1.21 if black)

Techniques for GFR estimation

Alternative clearance methods that use exogenous filtration markers, such as iothalamate sodium I 125 and ^{99m}Tc DTPA, are simpler, but are inconvenient and expensive, and require trained personnel. These are discussed in a later chapter.

- Cystatin—a 134-kDa protein, is produced by all nucleated cells at a relatively constant rate, unaltered by diet or inflammation. Preliminary studies show that serum cystatin is more sensitive and specific than serum creatinine for the estimation of GFR. A minor decrease in GFR will cause the cystatin levels to rise above normal while the serum creatinine is still within the normal range

- Serum creatinine—though it can provide a rough index of the level of GFR, it tends to overestimate GFR, particularly at low GFR. Because of the reciprocal relationship between clearance and serum creatinine, serum creatinine does not rise out of the normal range until there has been a substantial (50–70%) decrease in the GFR. However, in an individualized patient, a progressive increase in serum creatinine over time, even within the normal range, implies declining GFR. A significant disadvantage of using serum creatinine in isolation is that it is affected by a number of external factors, including renal failure, malnutrition, exercise, protein intake, drugs (e.g., cimetidine, trimethoprim, cephalosporins), and ketoacidosis. Therefore in clinical practice, the urinary clearance of creatinine is most commonly utilized

---

(e) CREATININE CLEARANCE

Normal values —85–135 mL/min (lower in females and the elderly)
  —children have similar values to adults

Introduction
- Creatinine is the non-enzymatic breakdown product of creatine and phosphocreatine (almost exclusively found in skeletal muscle)
- Daily production is constant in an individual, but physiological variations occur
- Mean creatinine production is higher
  - In men than in women
  - In younger than in older people
  - In blacks than in whites

Excretion is primarily by glomerular filtration, but is also secreted to a certain extent by the proximal tubules, thereby making it inferior to inulin as an ideal marker for GFR estimation. Thus creatinine clearance systematically overestimates GFR by about 10–20%, but this may be greater and more unpredictable in chronic renal failure.

Urine collection and analysis
- Patient should be advised to avoid a high protein intake 48 hours prior to sampling
- Ensure patient is well-hydrated
- Discard first morning void and then start urine collection for 24 hours
- After 24 hours patient to empty bladder one last time and save urine
- At the end of urine collection, a blood sample is taken for serum creatinine measurement
- Measure height and weight to calculate body surface area

The creatinine clearance is calculated using the following formula:

$$\text{Cr clearance} = \frac{\text{Urine conc of creatinine (mmol/L)} \times \text{Urine flow rate (mL/min)}}{\text{Plasma conc of creatinine (mmol/L)}}$$

Limitations
- Glomerular secretion of creatinine results in overestimation of GFR (cimetidine, trimethoprim, and pyrimethamine can inhibit secretory component)
- Inaccurate urine collection can yield incorrect results
- Artifacts can be caused by strenuous physical exercise or high protein intake prior to urine collection

---

- GFR (*abbreviated MDRD equation*) = 183 × (serum creatinine) − 1.154 × (age) − 0.203 × (0.742 if female) (×1.21 if black)
- Cr clearance overestimates GFR by about 10% to 20%
- $$\text{Cr clearance} = \frac{\text{Urine conc of creatinine (mmol/L)} \times \text{Urine flow rate (mL/min)}}{\text{Plasma conc of creatinine (mmol/L)}}$$

(f) 24-HOUR URINE FOR URINARY PROTEIN EXCRETION

Reference values
- Random urine dipstick   0–5 mg/dL—negative
  6–2,000 mg/dL—positive (trace to +2)
- 24-hour specimen   25–150 mg/24 h

Indications
- Significant proteinuria on dipstick analysis. Analysis of 24-hour urine specimen will help identify the cause of proteinuria
- Diagnosis of nephrotic syndrome (triad of edema, hypoalbuminemia, and proteinuria of >3 g/24 h)
- To assess prognosis of progressive disease—proteinuria is one of the most potent risk markers for renal function deterioration
- Aid diagnosis of multiple myeloma (immunoassay for Bence Jones protein)

Specimen collection and analysis
- No dietary restriction is required
- Discard first urine specimen; then save all urine for 24 hours in a refrigerated urine-collection bottle
- Send for analysis within 24 hours

Interpretation
Severity of proteinuria is best measured by quantifying absolute protein excretion (in 24 hours) rather than urinary protein concentration (influenced by dilution).

Normally—

- Low molecular weight proteins and small amounts of albumin are filtered, and then almost completely reabsorbed in the proximal tubule
- Net result is daily protein excretion of <150 mg (usually 40–80 mg), of which approximately 30% is albumin, 30% serum globulins, and 40% tissue proteins (primarily Tamm–Horsfall protein)

Previously, abnormal proteinuria was generally defined as the excretion of more than 150 mg of protein per day, but it is now clear that early renal disease is reflected by lesser degrees of proteinuria, particularly increased amounts of albuminuria.

Proteinuria can be classified by type and timing.

Timing
1. *Transient*: common in children, and following fever, exercise, and stress. Usually spontaneous resolution occurs within a few days.

2. *Intermittent:* commonly occurs in young males and related to postural changes. Excess proteinuria (<1 g/24 h) occurs in the upright position (due to increased renal vein pressure) but resolves in the recumbent position. Spontaneous resolution occurs in about 50%.

3. *Persistent:* is pathological and requires further evaluation to establish cause.

Type
1. *Glomerular*: (most common) is due to increased filtration (particularly albumin) across the glomerular capillary wall, and is a sensitive marker for the presence of glomerular disease. Proteinuria usually exceeds 1 g/24 h and can often be in excess of 3 g/24 h.

2. *Tubular*: interference with proximal tubular reabsorption, principally due to tubulointerstitial diseases (Fanconi's syndrome) can lead to increased excretion of smaller molecular weight proteins (rather than albumin). Tubular proteinuria is not diagnosed by dipstick analysis since low molecular weight proteins are not usually detected. Protein loss rarely exceeds 2–3 g/24 h but protein identification reveals *normal* proteins (cf. overflow proteinuria).

3. *Overflow*: increased excretion of *abnormal* low molecular weight proteins can occur with marked overproduction of a particular protein (almost always immunoglobulin light chains in multiple myeloma). Excretion of 300–2,000 mg of protein per 24 h is typical.

- Excellent, accurate, and cheap tool for protein excretion estimation
- Normal urinary protein excretion 25–150 mg/24 h
- Increased glomerular filtration of albumin most common cause of proteinuria
- Unable to identify the specific proteins—this requires protein electrophoresis or immunoassay

---

(g) 24-HOUR URINE ANALYSIS FOR STONE FORMERS

Overview
- Up to 75% of patients with an episode of urinary calculi will have a recurrence
- In the majority of recurrent stone formers, comprehensive medical evaluation, including urine tests, will identify dietary or metabolic factors predisposing them to stone formation
- While such extensive urine analysis may be considered time-consuming, instigation of appropriate therapy following urine analysis will help decrease subsequent costs and morbidity associated with recurrent nephrolithiasis

Objectives
- Identification of underlying physiological abnormality in recurrent stone formers
- Monitor efficacy of medical therapy in stone patients

24-hour urine collection

Accuracy of results escalates with an increase in the number of urine specimens analyzed and the length of period following stone passage. Samples should be collected when the patient is ambulatory rather than during in-hospital stay and at least 2 months after a stone event or stone intervention.

Ideally, patients should collect at least two 24-hour urine samples:

- One while remaining on their normal random diet (control urine)
- And a second following commencement of a standardized diet (standardized diet urine)

A standardized technique is as follows:

- Stop all medications which may interfere with metabolism of stone constituents for 1 week (e.g., calcium supplements, Vit C, Vit D, acetazolamide, phosphates, thiazides)
- Provide 2.5 L collecting bottles (with 10 mL of 5% thymol in isopropanol as preservative)
- Provide clear instructions to patient
  - Discard first voided morning sample—note time
  - Collect all urine thereafter in bottle for 24 hours
  - At exact start time collect the urine for last time
  - Analyze as soon as possible
  - Measure pH profile (test strips) throughout the day
  - If on random diet—record diet
- Commence on standardized diet for three days (to abolish or minimize dietary factors). On the fourth day, collect a 24-hour urine sample as described above

Identical or near identical abnormal urinary indices between the control and the standardized urine are indicative of metabolic disorders. If, however, abnormalities in the control urine are absent in the standardized sample, a dietary etiology is apparent (Table 1.7).

Cystinuria

- Inborn (autosomal recessive) metabolic disorder
- Excess excretion of the amino acids cystine, ornithine, lysine, and arginine
- Recurrent stone disease is common

TABLE 1.7. Reference range for 24-hour urine specimen

Urinary Variable	Normal Range	Comment
pH	5.8–6.8	Low urine pH (<5.8) promotes uric acid crystallization, but reduces citrate excretion Persistently elevated pH (secondary to ammonium and bicarbonate produced by urea-splitting organisms) is associated with struvite stone formation
Specific gravity	<1.010	Sufficient urine dilution is achieved with a urine production of >2 L/day
Volume	>2 L	Maintaining urine output of >2 L/24 h is the single most important therapeutic consideration Corresponds to fluid intake of 2.5–3 L/day
Calcium	<5 mmol	Over half the patients with recurrent stone disease will demonstrate increased calcium excretion Hypercalciuria defined as calcium excretion of >8 mmol/24 h Therapy (dietary or medical) justified if level >5 mmol/24 h
Uric acid	<4 mmol	Hyperuricosuria may be managed by a combination of diet (reduced purine content and increase fluid intake) and medication (allopurinol; citrate or bicarbonate to alkalinize urine)

TABLE 1.7. Continued

Urinary Variable	Normal Range	Comment
Citrate	>2.5 mmol	Citrate is a potent inhibitor of stone formation (by forming a soluble complex with calcium)
		Citraturia is increased in alkaline urine
		Management of hypocitraturia may be dietary (e.g., plants, alkalising drinks) or medical (e.g., potassium citrate)
Oxalate	<0.5 mmol	Hyperoxaluria may be primary (pyridoxine deficiency) or secondary (dietary excess or increased bioavailability in the gut)
		Increased oxalate absorption demonstrated in 44% of patients with calcium oxalate stones
Creatinine	15–20 mg/kg (females) 20–25 mg/kg (males)	Primary role of creatinine measurement is to assess completeness of urine collection
		Different collections in the same individual can be compared
Magnesium	>3.0 mmol	Magnesium inhibits stone formation by decreasing intestinal oxalate absorption
		May also complex with oxalate in urine
		Hypomagnesuria treated with magnesium supplements (200–400 mg/day)
Inorganic phosphate	<35 mmol	Hyperphosphaturia managed by dietary restrictions or by aluminium hydroxide (reduces intestinal absorption of phosphates)
Ammonium	<50 mmol	Ammonium excretion increased in the presence of infection with urea-splitting organisms
		Treatment includes eradication of bacteria and acidification of urine

- Urine dilution, dietary protein restriction, urine alkalization (to increase cystine solubility), and medical therapy are accepted treatment options

Reference range for 24-hour urine analysis for cystine:

- Normal   0.17–0.33 mmol
- Homozygous   >4.16 mmol
- Start treatment   <0.8 mmol
- Limit of solubility   1.33 mmol/L

Table 1.8 provides the reference range for urinary quantitative amino acid analysis in the adult patient.

- Indicated if recurrent and complicated stones
- Ideally two urine samples required (control/normal diet and standardized diet)

(h) URINARY ELECTROLYTES

- Urinary electrolyte concentration measurement is important in certain conditions
- There are, however, no fixed normal values
- Dietary intake and endogenous production of electrolytes can cause considerable variations even within the same individual
- Spot tests are of limited value
- Ideally a 24-hour urine specimen is used (plain container collection)

Reference range: 24-hour urine sample with a volume of 1.5–2.0 L (see Table 1.9)

I. Urinary sodium
- Normal range variable (between 20 and 400 mmol/day)
- Nearly totally dependent on dietary sodium intake
- Sodium excretion mainly by feces and urine

Indications
- Check compliance with low-salt diet in hypertensive patients
- In calcium-stone formers—reduction in Na^+ excretion improves hypercalciuria
- Cystine stone formers—cystinuria improves with a reduction in urine Na^+ excretion

TABLE 1.8. Reference range for urinary quantitative amino acid analysis in the adult patient

Amino Acid	Normal Range (μmol/mmol creatinine)
Cystine	3–7
Ornithine	0–5
Lysine	7–58
Arginine	0–5
Taurine	16–180
Aspartic acid	2–7
Threonine	7–29
Serine	21–50
Asparagine	0–23
Glutamic acid	0–12
Glutamine	20–76
Glycine	43–173
Alanine	16–68
Citrulline	0–4
A-aminobutyric acid	0–4
Valine	3–15
Methionine	5–21
Isoleucine	0–4
Leucine	2–11
Tyrosine	2–23
Phenylalanine	2–19
Homocystine	0
Histidine	26–153
Tryptophan	0

TABLE 1.9. Reference range: 24-hour urine sample (volume 1.5–2.0 liters)

Salt	mmol	mg
Sodium	<400	1,000–3,000
Potassium	25–125	500–1,500
Phosphate	50	500–1,100
Calcium	7–9	<200

In normal subjects—

- Urinary Na^+ excretion roughly equals average dietary intake
- Measurement of urinary Na^+ excretion can be used to check dietary compliance in patients with essential hypertension
- Restriction of Na^+ intake and adequate adherence should result in the excretion of less than 100 mmol/day
- Urine Na^+ concentration is a useful estimate of the patient's volume status

The kidneys, under the influence of the renin-angiotensin-aldosterone system, vary the rate of sodium (Na^+) excretion to maintain the effective circulating volume. Therefore, urine Na^+ concentration is a useful estimate of the patient's volume status and a urine Na^+ concentration below 20 mmol/L is generally indicative of hypovolemia. This finding is especially useful in the differential diagnosis of both hyponatremia and acute renal failure. The two major causes of hyponatremia are—

- Effective volume depletion
- Syndrome of inappropriate antidiuretic hormone secretion (SIADH)

Urine Na^+ concentration should be low in the former, but greater than 40 mmol/L in the SIADH, which is characterized by water retention but normal Na^+ handling (i.e., equal to intake). In acute renal failure secondary to acute tubular necrosis, urine Na^+ concentration usually exceeds 40 mmol/L due to a consequent inability to maximally reabsorb Na^+.

In patients with recurrent kidney stones, a 24-hour urine collection is typically obtained to determine if calcium or uric acid excretion is increased, both of which can predispose to stone formation. In general, Na^+ excretion above 75–100 mmol/day indicates that volume depletion is not a limiting factor for calcium or uric acid excretion.

The fractional excretion of sodium (FE_{Na}) gives an index of Na^+ reabsorption independent of changes in overall function and can be calculated as

$$\frac{\text{urine } Na^+ \times \text{serum creatinine}}{\text{serum } Na^+ \times \text{urine creatinine}} \times 100\%$$

An FE_{Na} of <1% is seen in pre-renal failure and >1% in acute tubular necrosis.

Limitations

A number of conditions can artificially alter urinary Na^+ concentration:

- A misleadingly low urine Na^+ concentration can be seen following renal ischemia, bilateral renal artery stenosis, or acute glomerulonephritis
- A falsely high rate of Na^+ excretion can occur with the use of diuretics, in aldosterone deficiency, or in advanced renal failure
- Urine Na^+ concentration is also influenced by the rate of water reabsorption

II. Urinary potassium

- Normal range variable (25–125 mmol/L)
- Potassium excretion varies with K^+ intake, response to aldosterone, changes in plasma K^+ concentration, acid–base balance, urine dilution, and sodium status

Indications

- Can aid in the diagnosis of unexplained hypokalemia

If K^+ depletion occurs, urinary K^+ excretion can fall to a minimum of 5–25 mmol/day. In comparison, the excretion of more than 25 mmol of K^+ per day indicates at least a component of renal K^+ wasting.

Measurement of K^+ excretion is less helpful in patients with hyperkalemia. If K^+ intake is increased slowly, normal subjects can take in and excrete more than 400 mmol of K^+ per day without a substantial elevation in the plasma K^+ concentration (normal daily intake is 40–120 mmol). Thus, chronic hyperkalemia must be associated with a defect in urinary K^+ excretion, since normal renal function would result in the rapid excretion of the excess K^+.

- *Causes of* **low** *urinary K^+ (<20 mmol/L) with hypokalemia:*
  —gastrointestinal loss (e.g., diarrhea, high output ileostomy, enterocutaneous fistula)
  —dietary deficiency
  —skin loss (e.g., burns)
- *Causes of* **high** *urinary K^+ (>20 mmol/L) with hypokalemia in normotensive patients:*
  —vomiting (urinary chloride will be low)
  —diuretic abuse

—renal tubular acidosis types 1 and 2 (K^+ wasting)

—diabetic ketoacidosis

- Causes of **high** urinary K^+ (>20 mmol/L) with hypokalemia in hypertensive patients:
  —hyperaldosteronism
  —mineralocorticoid excess

III. Urinary chloride

- No normal range but wide variation
- Mirrors urinary Na^+ excretion as chloride is reabsorbed and excreted with sodium throughout the nephron

Indications

- Aids diagnosis in unexplained normotensive hypokalemia

In hypokalemia,

- Cl^- low if hypokalemia caused by extra-renal NaCl or hydrogen chloride loss (e.g., diarrhea or vomiting)
- Cl^- high if hypokalemia caused by inappropriate loss of KCl (e.g., diuretic use)

(i) RENAL TUBULAR ACIDOSIS—ASSESSMENT OF URINARY ACIDIFICATION

Overview

- A urinary pH that never falls below 5.8 is suggestive of renal tubular acidosis (RTA)

The normal renal response to acidemia is to—

- Reabsorb all filtered bicarbonate
- Increase hydrogen excretion primarily by enhancing the excretion of ammonium ions in urine

Any inability of the renal tubules to perform these functions leads to a metabolic acidosis which typically—

- Is a normal anion gap (hyperchloremic) metabolic acidosis
- Occurs as a consequence of either net retention of hydrogen chloride or its equivalent (such as ammonium chloride) or the net loss of bicarbonate or its equivalent

There are three major subgroups of RTA with different clinical characteristics:

- Distal or type 1 RTA is characterized by an impaired capacity for hydrogen ion and therefore ammonium secretion. The impairment in hydrogen ion secretion is manifested as an abnormally high (>5.4) urine pH during systemic acidosis
- Proximal or type 2 RTA originates from the inability to reabsorb bicarbonate normally in the proximal tubule. Under normal conditions, virtually no bicarbonate is present in the final urine
- Hypoaldosteronism or type 4 RTA: impaired ammoniagenesis is the primary defect in type 4 RTA and is not discussed at any length in this book

RTA and nephrolithiasis from a urological perspective:

- Type 1 RTA is frequently associated with hypercalciuria, hyperphosphaturia, nephrolithiasis (with calcium phosphate or less often struvite stones), and nephrocalcinosis
- Up to 5% of all stone patients will have some form of type 1 RTA
- Metabolic acidosis promotes stone formation both by increased calcium and phosphate mobilization from bone and by direct reduction (via an unknown mechanism) of the tubular reabsorption of these ions
- Additional factors which encourage stone formation are the tendency of calcium phosphate to precipitate in alkaline urine and decreased excretion of citrate (inhibitor of stone formation)

Indications
- Unexplained hyperchloremic metabolic acidosis
- Assessment of recurrent stone formers

Diagnosis of type I renal tubular acidosis (*ammonium chloride loading test*)
This is the gold standard for the diagnosis of type I RTA.

Technique—

- Fast patient overnight
- Check urine pH and serum bicarbonate before commencing
- Urine pH < 5.4 suggests normal acidification ability and further tests are superfluous
- If serum bicarbonate low, and urine pH > 5.4, the diagnosis of RTA is confirmed

- Patient then given ammonium chloride capsules (dose 0.1 g/kg)
- Check urinary pH at hourly intervals for up to 8 hours (a consistent urine pH > 5.4 is diagnostic of RTA)
- After 3 hours following ammonium chloride, check venous bicarbonate levels to check for acidosis

---

(j) ADRENAL-SPECIFIC URINARY TESTS

Overview

Urinary assays for adrenal activity are generally restricted to measurement of steroid levels and catecholamine hormones or metabolites and reflect renal handling of the hormones. As a general rule, serum analysis is preferred, but urine assays can provide an integrated assessment of overall hormonal status. Due to the episodic release of adrenal hormones, random urine (or plasma) measurements can often be normal even in the presence of underlying pathology, and therefore a 24-hour specimen is mandatory.

Adrenal function

- Cortex—secretes cortisol, aldosterone, and androgens (dehydroepiandrosterone (DHEA), dehydroepiandrosterone sulphate (DHEAS) and androstenedione). Table 1.10 summarizes the normal reference values
  - Cortisol
    - 10% of circulating cortisol is free
    - 90% bound to serum proteins
    - Undergoes extensive modification during hepatic metabolism
    - Over 95% of cortisol is converted into soluble conjugated compound ready for urinary excretion
    - Only less than 1% of secreted cortisol is excreted unchanged in urine
  - Aldosterone
    - Up to 50% of circulating aldosterone is bound to serum albumin
    - Majority is deactivated by the liver
    - 5%–10% converted to aldosterone-18-glucoronide by the kidney
    - Only a small amount of free aldosterone is excreted in urine
  - Androgens
    - DHEA, DHEAS, and androstenedione are largely inactive, but are precursors for the active androgens testosterone and dihydrotestosterone

TABLE 1.10. Normal reference values for adrenal cortical hormones

Urinary Hormone	Normal Values (24-h urine)	Comment
Free cortisol	14–135 nmol/24 h or 5–50 μg/24 h (measured by high-performance liquid chromatography)	Less than 1% of cortisol is excreted in urine and therefore a significantly increased level of free urinary cortisol is virtually diagnostic of Cushing's syndrome; otherwise 24-hour urinary cortisol excretion is the most reliable index of cortisol secretion (*NB: false positives may occur during periods of increased cortisol secretion including stress (acutely ill, surgery, trauma and pregnancy)*)
Free aldosterone	>39 nmol/24 h or >14 μg/24 h	Elevated levels, in association with increased potassium loss (30 mmol/day) and an adequate sodium excretion (>200 mmol/day) are diagnostic of primary hyperaldosteronism
Aldosterone-18-glucoronide	14–56 nmol/24 h or 5–20 μg/24 h	Distinction between an aldosterone-producing adenoma and idiopathic hyperaldosteronism is not always possible but levels tend to be more elevated in the former (>42 μg/24 h, >126 nmol/24 h) than the latter (>25 μg/24 h, >70 nmol/24 h)
17-ketosteroids	17–52 μmol/24 h or 5–15 mg/24 h (females) 34–69 μmol/24 h or 10–20 mg/24 h (males)	Urinary 17-KS excretion is not an accurate test for the diagnosis of adrenal hyperandrogenism (compared to serum measurements); nevertheless, grossly elevated urinary 17-KS levels can be seen in adrenal carcinoma (as opposed to adenoma)

- Serum measurements are far superior to urinary measurements
- 17-ketosteroids (17-KS) excreted in urine (mainly consisting of DHEA, DHEAS, and their metabolites) are measured instead

Drugs which interfere with urinary assay include carbemazepine, spironolactone, tranquilisers, anti-epileptic medication, and antipsychotics and must be stopped for at least one week prior to assessment.

- Medulla
  - Secretes catecholamines (adrenaline and noradrenaline)
  - Catecholamines (<5%) and their metabolites (metanephrines and vanillymandelic acid) are excreted in urine
  - Excretion of these compounds is increased in the presence of a pheochromocytoma
  - Generally, small tumors release free catecholamines, whereas larger tumors are associated with higher levels of metabolites due to increased metabolization of the catecholamines within the tumor before release

In 10% of patients, increased urinary excretion of catecholamines and their metabolites will be secondary to essential hypertension. Although grossly elevated levels (at least twice normal) are diagnostic of pheochromocytoma, various drugs, foods, and medical conditions can alter the accuracy of the urinary results (see Table 1.11).

(k) URINARY MARKERS FOR TCC DETECTION

Overview
- Voided urine cytology (VUC) has been the standard non-invasive urinary marker for urothelial TCC detection
- VUC is cheap and relatively straightforward, but its intra-observer variability and poor sensitivity for TCC, especially low grade disease has limited its usefulness
- Numerous urinary biomarkers have been developed to help with early diagnosis, follow-up, prediction of tumor recurrence, progression, and clinical outcome
- Unfortunately none have shown either sufficient sensitivity or specificity, nor adequate efficacy in predicting outcome of TCC
- Urinary markers remain inferior to direct endoscopy

TABLE 1.11. Reference values for urinary catecholamines and their metabolites

Urinary Compound	Normal Levels	Causes of Inaccuracies
Adrenaline	<131 nmol/24 h or 24 µg/24 h	Levels may be increased by drugs (containing catecholamines, levadopa, labetalol, and anxiolytics), foodstuff (bananas, caffeine, peppers, alcohol), and conditions (surgery, trauma, stress, renal failure)
Noradrenaline	<591 nmol/24 h or 100 µg/24 h	
Metanephrine	<1,166 nmol/24 h or 230 µg/24 h	Levels increased by catecholamines and monoamine oxidase inhibitors
Normetanephrine	<2,738 nmol/24 h or 540 µg/24 h	
Vanillylmandelic acid	<35 µmol/24 h or 7 mg/24 h	Levels increased by catecholamines, levadopa, and foods containing vanillin
Homovanillic acid	48 µmol/24 h or 8.8 mg/24 h	Levels decreased by clofibrate, disulfiram, and monoamine oxidase inhibitors

- Point-of-care (POC) assays can be a useful adjunct to cystoscopy
- Virtually all urinary markers are superior to VUC with respect to sensitivity, but have a decreased specificity in the asymptomatic patient
- Urinary markers are not suitable for general screening for bladder cancer but may have a more defined role in the follow-up of patients with known bladder TCC

Indications
1. Investigation of hematuria
2. Surveillance of known bladder TCC—assess risk of recurrence
3. To predict risk of progression
4. To predict response to treatment
5. Non-invasive monitoring of upper tract disease

Although the United States Food and Drug Administration has approved several urine tests (e.g., BTA Stat, BTA TRAK, NMP22 tests) for the detection of tumor recurrence, whether any has sufficient diagnostic reliability to eliminate the need for cystoscopy is unclear. The common urinary markers are (see also Table 1.12)—

1. Bladder tumor antigen (BTA TRAK and BTA Stat)
2. Nuclear matrix protein (NMP22)
3. Fibrinogen degradation products (Accu-Dx)
4. Telomerase
5. Hyaluronic acid/hyaluronidase (HA-HAase test)
6. Immunocyt

(I) URINARY MARKERS FOR PROSTATE CANCER DETECTION

Overview
Measurement of serum prostate specific antigen (PSA) in its various forms still suffers from a lack of specificity in the detection of prostate cancer (CAP). Attention has therefore focused on the detection of cancer-specific gene markers in urine. The new urine based genetic test uPM3 assay detects the relative expression of the $DD3^{PCA3}$ (differential display code 3) gene within prostate cancer cells in urine.

TABLE 1.12. Common urinary markers

Marker	Function	Sensitivity (%) (range)	Specificity (%) (range)
BTA TRAK	Detects human complement factor H related protein Bladder tumor antigen Quantative	**66** (62–76)	**65** (51–98)
BTA Stat	Similar to BTA TRAK Qualitative POC assay Requires a few drops of urine	**70** (63–90)	**75** (52–93)
NMP22	Detects a nuclear mitotic apparatus protein abundant in TCC A POC assay available	**67** (44–100)	**78** (62–95)
Fibrinogen degradation factors	Detects urinary fibrinogen–fibrin degradation factors which are common in malignancy	**68** (50–86)	**86** (65–97)
Telomerase	Detects telomerase expressed by malignant cells Promising marker but requires laboratory analysis	**75** (55–86)	**86** (66–100)
HA-HAase	Detects hyaluronic acid and the enzyme that degradates it, hyalurinidase (both elevated in bladder cancer) Laboratory based assay	83	90
Immunocyt	Combines cytology with immunofluorescence assay detection of cancer related antigens and mucins Requires immunochemistry so not a POC assay Currently only a research tool	90	79

TABLE 1.13. Sensitivity and specificities of the uPM3 assay

PSA level (ng/ml)	Sensitivity (%)	Specificity (%)
<4	73	91
4–10	58	91
>10	79	80
Overall	**66**	**89**

- UPM3^{TM} is based on a specific gene PCA3
- PCA3 is over-expressed in prostate cancer tissue (average 34-fold, range 10–100-fold) compared to benign prostate tissue
- No other human tissues have ever been shown to produce PCA3.
- The DD3^{PCA3} gene is located at chromosome 9q21-22 and even minute amounts in urine can be detected using a nucleic acid amplification assay
- Following prostatic massage, the first 10–20 mL of urine is collected and tested for DD3^{PCA3}, which is over-expressed in 95% of CAP and therefore CAP-specific
- This is a relatively new test requiring specialized laboratory facilities and experience in a routine clinical setting is limited
- Detection depends on prostate cancer cells shed in the urine after prostate massage, which then need to be transported to the laboratory, resulting in potential loss of specimen quality
- Represents an exciting and promising non-invasive technique for the investigation of men with suspected CAP

The reported sensitivity and specificities of the uPM3 assay are as described in Table 1.13.

- UPM3 appears to be twice as specific as PSA for the detection of CAP, especially in men with a PSA <10 ng/L
- Up to 75% of men with a positive uPM3 test will go on have histological evidence of CAP following transrectal biopsy
- In addition, uPM3 seems to be a better predictor of outcome in patients undergoing a repeat prostate biopsy

Chapter 2
Blood Tests

(a) PROSTATE-SPECIFIC ANTIGEN (PSA)

Overview
PSA
- Is a 34-kilodalton (kDa) glycoprotein produced by the prostatic secretory epithelial cells which line the acini and the ducts of the prostate gland
- Is expressed in both benign and malignant prostatic conditions
- Is found in high concentrations in semen and is thought to cause liquefaction of the seminal coagulum
- Has a half-life of 3.2 days
- Is elevated in CAP and a variety of benign prostatic diseases (benign prostatic hyperplasia [BPH] and prostatic inflammation)
- Is organ-specific, but serum PSA levels cannot readily differentiate between various prostatic pathologies
- Has a limited specificity and sensitivity for CAP when used in isolation
- Nevertheless, forms the cornerstone of screening for CAP

Normally, the PSA prohormone (proPSA) is secreted into the lumen of the prostatic duct, where it is converted to the active form. A small proportion of the active PSA enters the blood circulation and is found bound to protease inhibitors such as 1-antichymotrypsin and alpha-2-macroglobulin. The remaining active PSA is converted to the inactive PSA form by proteolysis and is found circulating unbound in serum plasma (free PSA). The gene encoding for PSA is located on chromosome 19.

Indications
- Screening tool (in conjunction with digital rectal examination) for the detection of CAP. Annual examinations in men over 50

years of age, or from 40 years of age in high-risk groups (e.g., family history of CAP, African-American)
- Patients suspected of having CAP
- Surveillance and monitoring of CAP patients

Technique
- Patients must be counseled on the nature and implications of PSA testing (i.e., indications, possible need for further investigations such as prostate biopsies, and potential diagnosis of cancer)
- 5 mL of venous blood is required
- Record patient's age
- Age-specific PSA values are derived from commercial immunoassays based on monoclonal antibodies identification

Clinical implications
Normal values
Traditionally, PSA elevation above a cut-off reference value of 4.0 ng/mL has been regarded as abnormal and prostate biopsies are recommended. Since PSA increases with age, a single reference standard would appear inappropriate in men of all ages given that the clinical significance of CAP varies with increasing age. Moreover, though CAP is commoner with advancing age, there is a paradoxical gradual decrease in its clinical significance. Men of all ages do not have the same therapeutic aims. Therefore, attempts to improve the overall specificity and sensitivity, and decrease the number of false negative biopsies have resulted in the increased use of age-specific reference ranges (Table 2.1).

Factors affecting serum PSA
1. Age
Blood PSA concentration is dependent on patient age, and the increase in PSA with advancing age is attributable to a number of factors including—

- Normal hyperplasia of the aging prostatic epithelial cells
- A higher incidence of subclinical prostatitis
- The growing prevalence of microscopic, but clinically insignificant prostate cancer
- Areas of prostatic infarction
- Increased leakage of PSA into the serum

TABLE 2.1. Age-specific reference ranges

Age range (yr)	PSA (ng/mL)
40–49	0–2.5
50–59	0–3.5
60–69	0–4.5
70–79	0–6.5

2. BPH

More PSA per gram is produced by BPH (0.2 ng/mL of serum PSA per 1 g of BPH) than by normal prostatic tissue, making BPH the most common reason for mild elevations in serum PSA up to 10 ng/mL. The sensitivity of serum PSA ranges from 57% to 79% and specificity from 59% to 68% for CAP and in isolation, is insufficient to accurately distinguish between BPH and CAP. Therefore, within the range PSA 4–10 ng/mL, there is considerable overlap between men with BPH and early CAP, with the majority of patients requiring prostate biopsies to confirm histological diagnosis. Further elevations beyond this range are likely to suggest a malignant process.

3. CAP

The majority of prostate cancers express increased levels of PSA, making it the best available tool for the detection of and monitoring in patients with CAP. In 80% of patients with CAP, the PSA will increase sequentially. As a screening tool, it has a greater sensitivity than DRE though lacking in specificity. Nevertheless, serum PSA can in some instances be used to define percentage risk of CAP in patients (Table 2.2).

The utility of serum PSA in the staging and monitoring of patients with established CAP is discussed later in the chapter.

4. Prostatic inflammation/prostatitis

Both acute and chronic prostatitis can result in marked serum PSA elevations, with levels frequently estimated at >20 ng/mL. In patients with suspected prostatic inflammation and an elevated PSA, it is common clinical practice to treat patients with antibiotics and then repeat the PSA at least 6 weeks later, before proceeding to prostate biopsies. A significant decrease in PSA levels or a return to normal is suggestive of an inflammatory etiology. In addition, prostatic biopsies from such individuals often histologically confirm the presence of acute or chronic inflammation. It has been suggested that inflammation-mediated PSA

TABLE 2.2. The use of serum PSA to define percentage risk of CAP in patients

PSA Level (ng/mL)	Percentage Risk With a Negative DRE (%)	Percentage Risk With an Abnormal DRE (%)
<4	9	17
4–10	20–25 (consider biopsies)	45 (biopsies indicated)
>10	31–50 (biopsies indicated)	77 (biopsies indicated)

elevations result in a decreased free to total PSA ratio, but this is not a consistent finding.

5. Digital rectal examination
- Standard DRE may cause transient minor elevations in serum PSA which are not clinically significant
- The proportion of the transient rise may be greater in patients with a PSA of >20 ng/mL, but does not affect clinical management
- Prostatic massage, unless exceptionally vigorous, will produce clinically insignificant elevations in serum PSA in about 20% of patients
- There is no routine justification to delay PSA testing following DRE or prostate massage

6. Instrumentation
- Rigid and flexible cystoscopy will generate small rises in serum PSA, which may alter patient management
- Although some authors endorse the reliability of a post-cystoscopy PSA result, it is recommended that PSA testing be deferred by at least 4 weeks
- Transrectal ultrasound scan (TRUS) in isolation does not elevate results significantly, but post-biopsy testing should be deferred for a minimum period of 6 weeks
- Transurethral resection of the prostate (TURP) can cause abnormally increased serum PSA levels for up to 30 days, and a 6-week interval is recommended for a reliable result

7. 5-alpha-reductase inhibitors
Medications for BPH, such as finasteride and dutasteride, prevent the conversion of testosterone to the more potent dihydrotestosterone (DHT), by inhibition of 5-alpha-reductase. DHT levels are reduced by 60% after 6 months of treatment. The net impact is a 20% reduction in prostate volume with a simultaneous 50%

decrease in serum PSA levels after 6 months of therapy. This halving effect on PSA appears to be independent of patient age and initial aetiology of elevated PSA (i.e., BPH or CAP), and is reversed on withdrawal of treatment. It is important effectively to double the value of PSA results in patients on such therapy to obtain a truer reflection of the actual PSA level.

8. Others
Other forms of perineal trauma, such as prolonged bicycle or horse riding have been reported to elevate serum PSA, but the clinical implications are unclear. Ejaculation may cause minor, non-clinically-significant rises in PSA levels for two to three days, and some authors advocate sexual abstinence for three days prior to PSA testing, especially in young patients with a low PSA. While the passage of a urethral catheter may not significantly elevate serum PSA, acute and chronic urinary retention are well recognized influencing factors.

Modifications of PSA testing
1. PSA density
Larger prostate glands will produce more PSA. Therefore, in an attempt to resolve the considerable overlap in serum PSA between patients with BPH and early CAP, the notion of PSA density (PSAD) was introduced:

- PSAD = serum PSA divided by prostatic volume in mL (as estimated by TRUS)
- Traditional recommended cut-off of 0.15
- PSAD was not recommended in patients with a low (<4.0 ng/mL) or high (>20 ng/mL) PSA
- Presumed greatest utility in the 4–20 ng/mL PSA range, in terms of determining the need for prostate biopsies
- In the presence of a normal DRE, PSAD levels of <0.15 were said to be predictive of BPH, while levels of >0.15 were associated with a higher likelihood of a malignant pathology (and therefore proceeding to biopsies)

Unfortunately, PSAD has a number of shortcomings which preclude its widespread clinic use.

- A cut-off of 0.15 has a reasonable specificity (81%) but a disappointingly low sensitivity (52%), which would result in its missing almost half of the cancers

- In issues of decision-making, PSAD does not appear to have any significant advantage over age-specific PSA reference ranges
- The requirement of a TRUS-derived volume considerably elevates expense and discomfort to the patient
- Measurement inaccuracies can also result in wide variations on repeat testing, raising questions about the reproducibility of PSAD

For these above reasons, currently, PSAD is not routinely indicated in prostate cancer screening programmes or in the assessment of patients with suspected CAP.

2. PSA velocity

The assumption that a consistent upward trend in the serum PSA level is more likely to be secondary to a malignant process rather than BPH is the basis for the clinical usefulness of PSA velocity (PSAV).

- PSAV of >0.75 ng/mL per year has been shown correctly to distinguish patients with CAP from BPH with a sensitivity and specificity of 72% and 90%, respectively
- Some authors recommended at least three annual PSA estimations (by the same laboratory) in order to determine a representative PSAV

Overall, PSAV has been shown to be of limited value for a number of reasons.

- A cut-off value of 0.75 ng/mL per year is likely to result in a small but significant proportion of cancers being missed
- A patient with an abnormal age-specific PSA is likely to undergo biopsies at the earliest opportunity rather than wait for a whole year to enable PSAV calculation
- PSAV offers little additional benefit compared to the age-specific reference values, in patients undergoing screening programs for CAP

3. Molecular forms of PSA

The majority (90%) of serum PSA is complexed to 1-antichymotrypsin (PSA-ACT), while the rest is either free or bound to alpha-2-macroglobulin (PSA-AMG). Currently available assays can detect free and PSA-ACT, while immunoassays are as yet unable to detect PSA-AMG. It has been proposed that there is a lower concentration of free PSA in patients with CAP compared to those with BPH, such that there is a lower free:total (f/t) PSA ratio and a higher complexed:total (c/t) PSA ratio in prostate cancer patients.

There is much debate with regard to the role of ratios of molecular forms of PSA in decision-making in patients with PSA values between 4 and 10 ng/mL. The lower the f/t ratio, the better the specificity for CAP detection. Although various cut-off points have been proposed (e.g., 0.1, 0.19, and 0.25), patients with a ratio of <0.19 are usually referred for prostatic biopsy. In addition, there is some evidence to suggest that tumors with a lower f/t ratio are likely to be more aggressive.

Complexed PSA (and c/t PSA ratio) seems to outperform free PSA and f/t PSA ratio in predicting the likelihood of cancer. While this appears promising in increasing the sensitivity and specificity of PSA testing, the cut-off values have not been clearly defined and clinical utility therefore remains ambiguous.

PSA and cancer staging

In spite of the considerable overlap in serum PSA between stages of prostate cancer—

- PSA alone correlates reasonably well with pathological, and to a lesser extent, clinical CAP staging
- There is a direct relationship between tumor volume and serum PSA

Normograms (e.g., Partin's table) seek to enhance the predictive power of PSA by combining PSA with clinical stage and the histological (Gleason) grade in predicting the final pathological stage. These are now being used increasingly to direct patient management. As a general rule, the majority of men (80%) with CAP and a PSA of <4 ng/mL will have organ-confined disease on final analysis. The proportion of patients with extra-prostatic disease increases with a rising serum PSA level, with roughly 65% and <50% of patients having organ-confined disease with a PSA of 4–10 ng/mL and >10 ng/mL, respectively.

Lymph node metastases: multivariate analysis has demonstrated that PSA is the best predictor of the possibility of lymph node metastases, though its predictive ability is significantly enhanced if combined with clinical stage and Gleason grade. Nodal disease is—

- Rare in patients with PSA of <4 ng/mL
- Found in 20% of those with a PSA of >20 ng/mL
- Found in over 75% of patients with PSA >50 ng/mL

It is argued that use of predictive tables can significantly reduce the number of unnecessary lymph node sampling.

Skeletal metastases: PSA has also been shown to be the best individual predictor of results of a bone scan in patients with CAP. There is little justification in routinely performing bone scans in asymptomatic patients with a PSA <10 ng/mL, since the presence of skeletal metastases, based on a positive bone scan, is rare. The majority of patients with a significantly elevated PSA (>50 ng/mL) will have a positive bone scan.

- PSA has revolutionized detection and management CAP
- PSA remains the single most useful tumor marker compared to other cancers markers
- PSA shows good correlation with tumor stage, lymph node status, and likelihood of skeletal metastases
- Improvement in immunoassay detection techniques and modifications in the use of other molecular forms of PSA (e.g., free and complex PSA) may improve diagnostic accuracy
- Limitations:
  - Limited specificity and sensitivity
  - PSA affected by age, BPH, infection, lower urinary tract manipulation
  - <10% of CAP are non-PSA secreting
  - Widespread screening will inevitably result in over-investigation or over-treatment in a small proportion of patients

---

(b) ELECTROLYTES

Overview
- Electrolyte ions are critical for a variety of cellular reactions, including nerve impulse conduction and water balance
- Electrolyte imbalances may occur in virtually any urological pathological process
- Indications for electrolyte estimation are many and varied, and can be justified for almost any urological condition including—

- Existing or risk of renal failure
- Peri-operative (e.g., TURP, major surgery)
- In patients taking certain medications (e.g., diuretics, digoxin)
- Existing or risk of dehydration or malnutrition
- Urinary stone disease
- Organ failure (e.g., cardiac, liver, pulmonary failure)

Interpretation
Some urologically important causes of electrolyte disturbances are highlighted below (Table 2.3).

(c) TESTICULAR TUMOR MARKERS

Overview
Tumor markers are compounds produced by malignant neoplasms of the testis, which may be useful in the diagnosis and management of these tumors. Four markers have been described, although only the first three remain in clinical use:

- Beta human chorionic gonadotropin (βhCG)
- Alpha fetoprotein (AFP)
- Lactate dehydrogenase (LDH)
- Placental alkaline phosphatase (PALP)

Indications
- Diagnosis and management of suspected testicular tumors

Timing of evaluation
- Prior to radical orchidectomy
- Following radical orchidectomy or chemo-radiation
  - Weekly till levels back to normal
  - 2–3 monthly for the first 2 years
  - 6 monthly after the second year

Interpretation
Some of the basic characteristics of the tumor markers are described below (Table 2.4).

Diagnosis
Though tumor markers cannot replace orchidectomy and histological conformation in making the diagnosis of testicular malignancy, they provide strong support for a malignant diagnosis. Approximately 90% of patients with non-seminomatous germ cell tumors (NSGCT) will have elevated levels of either AFP or βhCG at the time of diagnosis. In addition, gross elevations

TABLE 2.3. Urologically important causes of electrolyte disturbances

Electrolyte	Normal Range (adults)	Levels Increased	Levels Decreased
Na^+	135–145 mmol/L	Is uncommon, but may occur in dehydration endocrine abnormalities (e.g., primary hyperaldosteronism, Conn's syndrome, Cushing's disease) Diabetes insipidus	Reflects a relative excess of body water rather than low total body sodium Causes include— • Excessive fluid loss (e.g., burns, diarrhea, vomiting) • Congestive cardiac failure • Excessive iv glucose infusion • Diuretics • TUR syndrome • Diabetic acidosis • Renal failure • Excessive ADH secretion
K^+	3.5–5.2 mmol/L	Renal failure (any aetiology) Trauma (e.g., burns, surgery, chemotherapy) K-sparing diuretics Metabolic acidosis Uncontrolled diabetes Endocrine (e.g., Addison's disease) Kidney transplant rejection	Diarrhea, vomiting, sweating Drugs (e.g., diuretics, steroids, insulin, penicillin) Starvation/malabsorption
Urea	3.0–8.8 mmol/L	Renal failure Dehydration	Pregnancy Hepatic failure
Creatinine	60–120 µmol/L	Renal failure Urinary obstruction	Pregnancy Small stature

Cl⁻	95–105 mmol/L	Dehydration Severe diarrhea Intestinal fistulae Respiratory alkalosis Primary hyperparathyroidism	Vomiting Diabetic ketoacidosis Renal tubular damage
Ca²⁺	(total) 2.1–2.65 mmol/L	Hyperparathyroidism Malignancy (metastases or PTH-producing tumors) Tuberculosis Excessive intake of milk, Vit D	Reduced albumin levels Hyperparathyroidism Hyperphosphataemia (renal failure) Malabsorption Drugs (e.g., bisphosphonates, cytotoxic drugs)
Uric acid	0.1–0.45 mmol/L	Gout Renal failure Alcoholism Hypothyroidism Obesity Diet (e.g., purine rich—liver, kidney)	Fanconi's syndrome Aspirin Diet (e.g., tea, coffee)
Urate	(males) <420 μmol/L (females) <360 μmol/L	Drugs (e.g., alcohol, aspirin, cytotoxic drugs, frusemide) Diet (e.g., anchovies, kidney, liver)	Drugs (e.g., allopurinol) Hepatitis

Muscle disease
Congestive cardiac failure
Shock
Dehydration
Rhabdomyolysis

Decreased muscle mass
Advanced hepatic failure
Poor dietary protein

TABLE 2.4. Basic characteristics of testicular tumor markers

Marker	Comment	Normal	Half-Life	False Positives
βhCG	Normally a product of the placenta β subunit of hCG is measured βhCG most commonly elevated tumor marker in testicular cancer Levels >10,000 mIU/mL only seen in NSGCT	<5 mIU/mL	24–36 h	Hypogonadal state Marijuana Pituitary secretion of βhCG
AFP	Normally produced by the fetal yolk sac and other organs Not produced by seminomas Levels >10,000 ng/mL only seen in NSGCT and hepatocellular cancer	<5 ng/mL	5 days	Hepatocellular tumors Gastrointestinal tumors Hepatic damage (e.g., cirrhosis, hepatitis) Drug or alcohol abuse
LDH	Normally found in muscle, liver, heart, kidney, brain May be only marker elevated in seminoma Correlates with tumor burden Poor specificity Five isoenzymes (LD1 most testis specific)	100–190 IU/L <1.5 times upper limit of normal <109 IU/L (for LD1)	2.8 days	May be produced by virtually any tumors Myocardial infarction, cardiac failure, anemia, pulmonary embolism Hemolysis of blood sample
PALP	Isoform of alkaline phosphatase May be more sensitive in seminoma	<100 KAU/L		Other malignancies (e.g., lung, pancreas, stomach, colon, and ovary) Smoking

TABLE 2.5. Histological tumor sub-types associated with elevations in specific markers

Tumor type	Cases with abnormal βhCG (%)	Cases with abnormal AFP (%)	Cases with abnormal LDH (%)
Seminoma	5–10	0–2	30–80
Teratoma	25	38	60
Teratocarcinoma	57	64	
Embryonal	60	70	
Choriocarcinoma	100	0	

(>10,000 units) in these markers are rarely found in men except in NSGCT.

Furthermore, levels of AFP and βhCG do correlate with the clinical stage of the disease. Elevated levels of βhCG in seminoma and AFP in NSGCT increase from approximately 10% in stage I disease to 30–60% in disseminated disease. Histological tumor subtypes are associated with elevations in specific markers (see Table 2.5).

Prognostic value

The International Germ Cell Cancer Collaborative Group (IGCCCG) have now included serum levels of testicular markers as independent prognostic indicators, and three risk categories have been identified:

1. Good prognosis
   - NSGCT
     - AFP <1,000 ng/mL
     - βhCG <5,000 mIU/mL
     - LDH <1.5 times upper limit of normal
   - Seminoma
     - Normal AFP
     - Any level of βhCG or LDH

2. Intermediate prognosis
   - NSGCT
     - AFP 1,000–10,000 ng/mL
     - βhCG 5,000–50,000 mIU/mL
     - LDH 1.5–10 times upper limit of normal
   - Seminoma
     - Normal AFP
     - Any level of βhCG or LDH

3. Poor prognosis
   - NSGCT
     - AFP >10,000 ng/mL
     - βhCG >50,000 mIU/mL
     - LDH >10 times upper limit of normal

Following therapy, the levels of elevated tumor markers should fall at a rate in keeping with the respective half-lives. Patients in whom the serum marker levels fail to decline rapidly, never reach normal, or increase, are more likely to have one or more of the following:

a) Residual disease
b) Poor response to treatment
c) Requirement of early salvage therapy

The time taken for normalization of markers should be—

- βhCG—2 weeks
- LDH—2 weeks
- AFP—4 weeks

Should the marker levels remain elevated following orchidectomy, further cross-sectional imaging must be undertaken as this often indicates systemic metastatic disease rather than nodal disease. It is also noteworthy that up to 20% of men with normalized tumor marker levels post-therapy may still have residual microscopic disease.

Rising tumor marker levels following systemic treatment—

- Is a poor prognostic indicator and is usually due to active disease
- A rising βhCG represents increasing cancer burden and in such situations, radiological confirmation of recurrent disease may often lag behind increased marker activity by a few months
- A rising LDH is indicative of relapse. It is important to exclude any other causes of false-positive results prior to initiating therapy

LD1 isoenzyme of LDH
Recent evidence has suggested that LD1 may be a useful tumor marker in the management of testicular germ cell tumors based on certain observations.

- In patients with seminoma, LD-1 is elevated more often AFP and βhCG
- In metastatic disease, LD1 appears to be a superior prognostic marker than serum LDH
- LD1 is a better predictor of relapse in patients with non-seminomatous germ cell tumors compared to the other tumor markers
- LD1 reflects a typical chromosomal abnormality noted in patients with germ cell tumor of the testis (high copy number of 12p chromosome)

Serum measurement of LD1 isoenzyme of LDH appears to be a promising testis tumor marker, but further studies are required before it is established in routine clinical practice.

(d) BONE DISEASE RELATED TO UROLOGY

Overview
Certain urological conditions may have a direct impact on skeletal activity and calcium metabolism. Most of the body calcium and phosphate is tightly packed in bones and serum calcium levels and is kept constant by a complex interaction between vitamin D, parathyroid hormone (PTH), and calcitonin. Alkaline phosphatase (ALP) levels increase with abnormal osteoblastic activity in bone. Some common examples of interactions between bone disease and urological conditions include—

- Renal calculi and hypercalcemia–hyperparathyroidism, metastatic bone disease
- Androgen deprivation for prostate cancer and osteoporosis
- Effects of chronic renal failure (CRF) on bone mineralisation

Normal reference range is presented in Table 2.6.

Hypercalcemia
The renal effects of hypercalcemia include an increased glomerular filtration of calcium (hypercalciuria) as well as increased urinary phosphate excretion. The urological effects of these include—

- Renal stone formation
- Nocturia/polyuria—due to decreased concentrating effects of the renal tubule, secondary to hypercalciuria

TABLE 2.6. Normal reference range for markers of bone activity

Serum Levels	Normal Range
Calcium	2.2–2.6 mmol/L
Phosphate	0.8–1.45 mmol/L
PTH	10–65 ng/L
ALP	90–300 IU/L

Urological patients with hypercalcemia must be investigated for possible causes, which include—

- Excess PTH—primary (pituitary adenoma) or tertiary (secondary to renal failure)
- Malignant disease (most common cause of hypercalcemia in the in-patient setting)—bone metastases from prostate, kidney, etc. Hypercalcemia may be due to direct destruction of bone or production of a bone-resorption substance called PTH related polypeptide
- Excess Vit D—iatrogenic or self-administered; sarcoidosis
- Drugs—thiazides
- Others—"milk alkali" syndrome, immobility

Osteoporosis
- Castration, either medical (LHRH analogue) or surgical can cause a reduction of up to 17% in the bone mineral density in patients over 3 years
- Maximum loss occurs within the first year of treatment
- May lead to an increased incidence of osteoporosis and subsequent osteoporotic fractures
- Recommended that all patients commencing on androgen deprivation therapy should undergo surveillance checks on bone mineral density starting at 1 year onwards

Osteoporosis is not a disease of calcium metabolism and therefore serum calcium, phosphate, and ALP are often within normal limits. Ideally patients should undergo—

- Bone mass evaluation (DXA—double x-ray absorptiometry) scan
- Measurement of urinary NTx (type 1 collagen N-telopeptides), a bone marker for resorption suggesting increased bone turnover

TABLE 2.7. Trends in serum bone markers in pathological conditions

Condition	Calcium	Phosphate	ALP	PTH
Hyperparathyroidism	H	L	N,H	H
Malignancy related Hypercalcemia	H,N	L,N	H	N,L,H
Osteoporosis	N	N	N	N
Osteomalacia	N,L	N,L	H	N

(H = high; N = normal; L = low)

Osteomalacia

- CRF results in inadequate conversion of 25-hydroxy-Vit D to the more potent 1,25-dihydroxy-Vit D, and therefore results in insufficient mineralization of the osteoid framework
- Results in soft bones, bone pain, and pathological fractures
- Serum bone markers may be normal and the diagnostic gold standard remains the bone biopsy

In conclusion, Table 2.7 highlights certain trends in serum values of the common bone markers in pathological conditions.

(e) SEX HORMONE PROFILE

Overview

An understanding of the hypothalamic–pituitary–gonadal axis is vital for the management of men with infertility and erectile dysfunction (ED). The commonly encountered hormones include—

- LHRH—luteinizing hormone releasing factor
- LH—luteinizing hormone
- FSH—follicle-stimulating hormone
- Prolactin
- Testosterone

Pulses of LHRH from the hypothalamus stimulate LH and FSH release from the anterior pituitary.

- LH stimulates testosterone production from Leydig cells of the testis
- FSH stimulates Sertoli cells in the seminiferous tubules to produce mature sperm
- Production of inhibin is increased by FSH release, and this effects a negative feedback to the pituitary to decrease FSH release

Testosterone acts—

- Locally (within the testis to aid spermatogenesis)
- Systemically (to produce male secondary sexual characteristics, anabolism, and libido)
- To have a negative feedback on the hypothalamus/pituitary to inhibit LHRH secretion.

Prolactin (produced by the anterior pituitary)—

- Role in men not completely understood
- Thought to increase concentration of LH receptors in Leydig cells (and therefore increase testosterone levels)
- Enhances the effects of testosterone and helps maintain libido

Table 2.8 highlights some of the common features related to sex hormones in males.

Indications for male hormonal evaluation
- Investigation of ED (if symptoms of impotence and low libido)
- Investigation of infertility (if sperm concentration <10 million sperm/mL on semen analysis)
- Signs/features of endocrine abnormality

Interpretation
Hormonal profile assessment may help identify specific endocrine abnormalities (Table 2.9).

(f) SERUM MARKERS OF ADRENAL FUNCTION

Overview
A basic review of the adrenal steroids hormones is provided in the chapter on urinary adrenal markers (Chapter 1i). A number of serum-based investigations can be applied in the investigation of adrenal malfunction:

- Adrenal cortex secretes—
  - Aldosterone (mineralocorticoid)—release is mainly controlled by the renin-angiotensin system
  - Cortisol (glucocorticoid)
  - Androgens (dehydroepiandrosterone [DHEA], dehydroepiandrosterone sulphate [DHEAS] and androstenedione)

Hormone	Normal serum levels	Half-Life	Levels elevated by—	Levels decreased by—
LHRH		5–7 min	Prostaglandins	Sex hormones—testosterone FSH, LH Opioids Hypothalamic failure
LH	1.42–15.4 IU/L	30 min	Hypogonadism Testicular feminisation syndrome Testicular failure Anorchia	Pituitary failure Hypothalamic failure (Kallmann's syndrome)
FSH	1.24–7.8 IU/L	240 min	Turner's syndrome Hypogonadism Testicular failure Anorchia Hypopituitarism Castration Alcoholism	Pituitary failure Hypothalamic failure Some adrenal or testis cancers
Testosterone	9–38 nmol/L	1–12 days	Hyperthyroidism Adrenal tumors Androgen resistance Anti-androgens Estrogens	Hypogonadism Klinefelter's syndrome Orchidectomy Hypopituitarism Cirrhosis LHRH analogs
Prolactin	<20 µg/L	20 min	Prolactin-secreting pituitary tumors Acromegaly	Pituitary apoplexy Kallmann's syndrome

TABLE 2.9. Trends in serum hormone levels for specific endocrine abnormalities

Endocrine Abnormality	Testosterone	LH	FSH	Prolactin
Normal or obstructive azospermia	Normal	Normal	Normal	Normal
Testicular failure	Low	Normal/ high	High	Normal
Isolated spermatogenic failure	Normal	Normal	High	Normal
Kallmann's syndrome (hypogonadotrophic hypogonadism)	Low	Low	Low	Normal
Hyperprolactinaemia	Low	Low	Low/ normal	High
Androgen resistance	High	High	High	Normal

Cortisol and androgen secretion is dependent on circulating adrenocorticotrophic hormone (ACTH) from the pituitary. All these hormones are subject to diurnal variations, as well as changes in response to factors such as stress and injury. Therefore random estimations of serum hormones are of limited use.

- Adrenal medulla—secretes catecholamines (adrenaline and noradrenaline) and is controlled by the hypothalamus and sympathetic nervous system

Adrenal disease may include—

- Adrenal insuffiency/hypoadrenalism—e.g., Addison's disease
- Glucocorticoid excess—e.g., Cushing's syndrome
- Hyperaldosteronism—e.g., Conn's syndrome
- Catecholamine excess (e.g., pheochromocytoma)

Serum-based tests for the diagnosis of—

1. Hypoadrenalism—e.g., Addison's disease (Table 2.10)
2. Glucocorticoid excess—e.g., Cushing's syndrome (Table 2.11)
3. Hyperaldosteronism—e.g., Conn's syndrome (Table 2.12)
4. Catecholamine excess (e.g., pheochromocytoma)

TABLE 2.10. Serum based tests for the diagnosis of hypoadrenalism

Serum Tests	Comments
FBC	Often a lymphocytosis and oesinophilia
Electrolytes	Hyperkalemia, hyponatremia (due to ↓ mineralocorticoid) ↑ Urea, ↑ calcium, ↑ LFTs Hypoglycemia
Hormones	Cortisol levels low—<100 nmol/L (random measurements of little use) Aldosterone may be low (normal range 111–860 pmol/L) ACTH level >80 ng/L
Short ACTH (synacthen test)	Tetracosactide 250 μg given im or iv at time 0 Measure plasma cortisol at time 0, 20, and 60 min A normal response should show cortisol increase to >550 nmol/L
ACTH (synacthen test)	Depot tetracosactide 1 mg at time 0 Plasma cortisol measurement at time 0 and 1, 2, 3, 4, 5, 8, and 24 h Normal response is a cortisol rise of >550 nmol/L (max > 1,000 nmol/L)

TABLE 2.11. Serum based tests for the diagnosis of glucocorticoid excess

Serum Tests	Comments
Midnight cortisol level	Levels > 200 nmol/L (between 2300 and 0100 h) indicates loss of diurnal rhythm
Dexamethasone suppression	1 mg dexamethasone before bed at 2300 h Measure plasma cortisol at 0900 h Levels of <100 nmol/L exclude Cushing's disease

TABLE 2.12. Serum based tests for the diagnosis of hyperaldosteronism

Serum Tests	Comments
Electrolytes	Hypokalemia
Hormones	Aldosterone will be high (normal range 111–860 pmol/L) Serum renin will be low (<1.9 ng/mL/h)
Saline suppression test	Normal saline infusion (300 mmol over 4 h) Lack of suppression (high serum aldosterone) is diagnostic of hyperaldosteronism

Collection of 24-hour urine samples for catecholamine metabo-lites is the best method of diagnosis of catecholamine excers as in pheochromocytoma (see Chapter 1i), but elevated levels of serum adrenaline and noradrenaline taken after 30 minutes' rest can also prove useful.

Normal serum levels at rest are—

- Adrenaline <600 pmol/L
- Noradrenaline 0.41–4.43 nmol/L

Chapter 3
Radiology

(a) PLAIN ABDOMINAL RADIOGRAPH (KUB)

Overview
- Plain KUB incorporates the entire urinary tract—kidneys, ureter, and bladder (KUB)
- Upper limit lies above the adrenal glands, while the inferior limit lies just below the symphysis pubis

Indications
- Diagnosis of calcium-containing renal tract calculi (Fig. 3.1a)
- Control (scout) film prior to contrast administration
- Assess efficacy of stone treatment (e.g., shockwave lithotripsy)
- Check position and status of ureteric stents and foreign bodies/devices in the urinary tract (Fig.3.1b)
- In addition, a KUB will demonstrate intestinal gas patterns and certain soft tissue abnormalities

Technique and radiation
- Antero-posterior (AP) full-length view in full expiration
- Lateral films may be required to clarify the position of certain calcifications
- Bowel preparation prior to test will improve image quality and yield, but is not mandatory

Effective radiation dose is 1.5 mSv (equivalent to 9 months of background radiation or 3,750 miles traveled by car).

Interpretation
Appropriate interpretation requires a systematic approach.

- Firstly, the renal tract and its anatomical markings are scrutinized

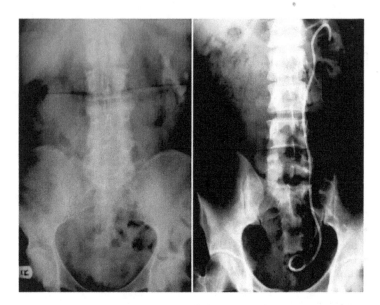

FIGURE 3.1. KUB showing a partial left renal staghorn stone (**left**) and a left ureteric stent (**right**) (Courtesy of Dr A Bradley, Wythenshawe, Manchester)

- Other intraabdominal and pelvic organs are identified
- Abnormal intestinal gas pattern is usually obviously apparent
- Look for bony abnormalities in the spine and bony pelvis

Renal tract
- Kidneys—renal hilum moves with respiration but tends to lie at the level of L2 lumbar vertebrae. The size (usually 11–13 cm in adults), shape, and position of both kidneys should be observed
- Ureters—the ureteric line is traced inferiorly, along the tip of the transverse processes of the lumbar vertabrae, over the sacroiliac joint, then lateral within the bony pelvis towards the ischial spine before sharply turning medially to enter the bladder. Note any calcifications—but non-urinary calcification can often confound matters

Causes of abnormal calcification on KUB include—

- Renal tract calculi (70–90% are radio-opaque and visible on KUB. Stones smaller than 1–2 mm may be missed)

- Calcified lymph nodes (common in the elderly)
- Phleboliths (very common in the pelvis)
- Calcified costal cartilages
- Renal nephrocalcinosis (seen in hyperparathyroidism, renal tubular acidosis, and medullary sponge kidneys)
- Aortic calcifications
- Prostatic calcification (can be seen in chronic prostatitis)
- Adrenal calcification
- Parenchymal calcification within cysts or tumors
- Calcified uterine fibroids
- Tuberculosis of the kidney

Soft tissue abnormalities—It is possible to assess the outline—and therefore the shape, size, and displacement—of organs such as the kidneys, liver, spleen, and bladder. Absence of psoas shadow may suggest a retroperitoneal mass or fluid collection.

Abdominal gas pattern—A plain film is invaluable in the diagnosis of intestinal obstruction (with bowel dilatation proximal to the level of obstruction) and ileus. Gross fecal loading can be easily verified.

Bony abnormalities—A systematic examination of the lower vertebral column may reveal fractures or obvious bony metastases, as well as provide evidence of neurological disease, including spina bifida and sacral agenesis. Metastases to the bony pelvis is common and can be seen on the KUB film.

Advantages

The KUB film is an invaluable tool in the assessment of urinary tract disease and has a number of distinct advantages:

- Cheap
- Non-invasive
- Will easily identify high-density calcified stones (calcium oxalate, calcium phosphate) as well as low-density struvite and cystine stones
- Small radiation dose, therefore can be repeated
- Provides useful information about abdominal organs and intestinal obstruction

Drawbacks

- Misses up to 30% of stones (e.g., radiolucent stones such as uric acid and cystine, stones with low calcium content, and small stones)

- Can be difficult to distinguish between calcification within and outside the renal tract
- Bowel gas and fecal loading can obscure small calcifications

---

(b) INTRAVENOUS UROGRAPHY (IVU)

Overview
- IVU (or IVP—intravenous pyelography) provides anatomical, as well as functional, information
- Iodine-containing intravenous contrast medium is filtered and excreted by the kidneys, thereby providing excellent opacification of entire renal tract
- CT scanning is replacing the use of IVU in many urological conditions

Indications
- Investigation and surveillance of urinary stone disease (Fig. 3.2a–c)
- Investigation of hematuria (to exclude upper tract tumors)—(Fig. 3.2d)
- Investigation of upper tract obstruction (although ultrasound and radionucleotide studies are commonly used)
- Assessment of anatomical abnormalities (duplications and anomalies)
- Assessment of renal disease (e.g., medullary sponge kidneys, papillary necrosis, renal scarring, and renal tuberculosis)
- Management of renal tract trauma (in certain conditions, such as on-table IVU)

Technique and radiation
- Contraindicated in pregnant patients and those with a history of intravenous contrast allergy
- Fluid restriction is not required with modern low osmotic media
- Bowel preparation while desirable, is not mandatory
- Control KUB film is taken to identify any areas of calcification which may be obscured later by contrast
- 50 mL to 100 mL of contrast medium (1 mL/kg body weight of 300 mg of iodine per mL of solution) is injected into the antecubital vein using an 18-gauge cannula

Sequence of films post-contrast injection (all films AP view):

- *Immediate film*: within 1 minute of injection (arm to kidney time is approx 15 seconds). This demonstrates the nephrogram

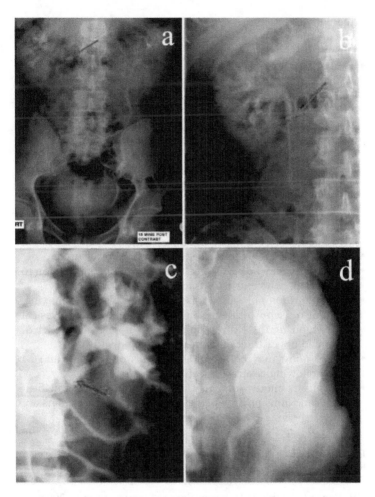

FIGURE 3.2. IVU showing partially obstructing right upper ureteric calculus at (**a**) 15 and (**b**) 30 minutes following contrast; (**c**) complete obstruction due to left proximal ureteric stone and (**d**) tomogram showing TCC renal pelvis and lower pole infundibulum and calyces (Courtesy of Dr A Bradley, Wythenshawe, Manchester)

(contrast in the renal tubules) which will be dense in the presence of obstruction. After a delay of 2–3 min, contrast enters the collecting system and reveals the pyelogram. Some radiologists recommend up to three tomographic views during the immediate phase at the level of a third of the AP diameter of the patient (~8–12 cm) to provide easier identification of renal calcification and masses. Tomography is not routinely used now. If such details are needed CT is usually preferred

- *5-min film*: this demonstrates the full pyelographic phase with visualization of the collecting system and the proximal (and sometimes distal) ureter. The sequence of further films is determined by this film. Note any dilatation (suggestive of obstruction/stasis) and filling defect (peristalsis, tumors, stones). A compression band applied at the level of the anterior superior iliac spines (corresponding to the ureters crossing over the pelvic brim) will produce better pelvicalyceal filling. Avoid compression if—
  - i. Abdominal trauma
  - ii. After recent renal surgery
  - iii. In the presence of a large abdominal mass
  - iv. In demonstrable upper tract obstruction
- *15-min film*: may be performed to show the lower ureter
- *Release film*: may be performed after release of compression to visualize the whole urinary tract
- *Post-micturition film*: allows assessment of bladder emptying, but is also useful in diagnosing bladder tumors, juxtavesical stones, and urethral diverticulum. Also note if any relief of presumed upper tract dilatation following micturition
- *Delayed films*: may be useful at intervals of 1, 4, 12, and 24 hours following contrast injection if obstructed
- *Other films*: oblique views may help clarify location of calcification. Prone films provide better ureteric filling. Erect films are best for showing renal ptosis and cystoceles

Effective radiation dose is 4.6 mSv (equivalent to 2.5 years of background radiation or 11,500 miles traveled by car).

NB: For an on-table IVU, larger doses of contrast (up to 200 mL) are frequently required. A combination of poor intra-operative renal perfusion and inadequate bowel preparation usually results in poor images. Most commonly a single film is taken 10 minutes following the contrast injection, but a sequence of films can be performed at 1, 5, 15, and 30 minutes.

Interpretation
The IVU is best interpreted as it is being performed to allow modification of technique. A systematic approach is recommended.

Check for two functioning kidneys, as well as their size, shape (horse-shoe?), contours (renal masses), and cortical thickness (usually a marker for renal function). The renal pelvis and calyces must be examined for adequate filling (filling defects?), distortion (mass effect from a space-occupying lesion), duplication, and distension (suggestive of obstruction). The features of an obstructed upper urinary tract include—

1. Dense nephrogram
2. Delayed pyelogram
3. Distension of the collecting system of ureter above level of obstruction
4. Contrast extravasation

A dense nephrogram may also be noted in patients with renal vein thrombosis and renal artery stenosis (delayed nephrogram), but the subsequent pelvicalyceal distension seen in renal tract obstruction, is absent.

The ureters may demonstrate filling defects, duplications, distension, and stricture formation. Calcification seen on the control film can be confirmed to be within or outside the renal tract.

Common bladder abnormalities have been discussed earlier. Although visualization of the lower urinary tract is often sub-optimal using IVU, it may be used for further information on urethral anatomy or as a micturition study when the retrograde approach is not possible.

IVU in children
- Has been largely replaced by USS, CT scanning, and nuclear medicine studies
- Still useful in children with complicated stone disease, abnormal/variant upper tract anatomy, and hematuria
- Certain modifications are required:
  - Limit amount of contrast (1 mL/kg body weight)
  - Limit number of films to three
  - Avoid dehydration
  - Avoid bowel preparation
  - Avoid compression

Advantages
- Prompt visualization of entire urinary tract with good demonstration of anatomy

- Excellent demonstration of renal tract calculi (>90%)
- Functional assessment of obstruction (high or low grade)
- Qualitative assessment of overall kidney function (degree of opacification, cortical thickness)
- Can be performed/interpreted by non-radiologists
- Cheap

Drawbacks
- Requires intravenous access
- Requires contrast (see below for *Contrast-related adverse effects*)
- Use of radiation
- Dependant on renal function (images poor if serum creatinine >200 µmol/L)
- May miss renal masses if not in line of renal contour
- Unable to distinguish between solid and cystic renal masses
- Cannot provide accurate estimation of renal function

Intravenous contrast media and the kidneys
IVU requires the administration of contrast media (CM), which possess intrinsic toxicity. The media may be—

- High-osmolar contrast media (HOCM) or
- Low osmolarity (LOCM)
- Ionic or
- Non-ionic

The toxicity of CM is a function of its osmolarity, chemical structure (chemotoxicity), and lipophilicity. The toxic effects may be chemotoxic (affect any organ system) or be idiosyncratic (anaphylactoid). A review of the potential widespread adverse effects of CM is not within the scope of this section; therefore, only nephrotoxic changes will be addressed in the table below (Table 3.1).

Metformin and contrast-related nephrotoxicity
Metformin accumulates in the kidneys if renal excretion is impaired following contrast injection and can therefore cause lactic acidosis, further aggravating the renal insult. Preexisting renal insuffiency, dehydration, and continued use of metformin (in the presence of renal impairment) are the main risk factors. The European Society of Urogenital Radiology guidelines have been summarized below (Table 3.2).

TABLE 3.1. Contrast media related toxicity

	Nephrotoxic Effects	Idiosyncratic (anaphylactoid) Effects
Incidence	~5% for LOCM ≦20% with HOCM	Mild (~3.5%) Moderate (LOCM 0.2%, HOCM 1%) Severe (LOCM 0.04%, HOCM 0.1%)
Features	↓ creatinine clearance ↑ serum creatinine (>25% or 44 mmol/L) Deterioration peaks within 3–4 days, but usually returns to normal within 2 weeks Oligouria Renal failure	(Independent of dose and concentration of CM) Mild—altered taste, nausea, vomiting, warm feeling, urticaria Moderate—severe vomiting, fainting, severe urticaria, facial and laryngeal edema, bronchospasms (usually require treatment) Severe (requires immediate intervention)—shock, pulmonary edema, cardio-respiratory arrest, convulsions, and death
Risk factors	*Patient factors* Preexisting renal impairment (present in 90% of patients with nephrotoxicity) Diabetes mellitus (27% to 75% of patients will develop renal impairment. In half of these, impairment will be permanent) Concurrent drugs such as gentamicin, cisplatin, non-steroidals (stop for 24h prior) Patient age (>70 years) *Contrast media factors* Dose (positive correlation between dose and rise in serum creatinine)	HOCM have increased risk Previous history of reaction to CM (fourfold increase in risk) Minor risk factors include a history of asthma, hay-fever and food allergies

TABLE 3.1. *Continued*

	Nephrotoxic Effects	Idiosyncratic (anaphylactoid) Effects
Mechanism	LOCM better than HOCM Intra-arterial injection has greater risk Reduction in renal perfusion Adverse cardio-toxic effects ↑ peripheral vasodilation ↓ renal blood flow Dehydration Osmotic diuresis Tubulo-glomerular injury Direct chemotoxic effect Impaired perfusion Hyperosmolar effects Internal obstructive uropathy Vacuolation of tubular cells Precipitation of Tamm–Horsfall protein	Simulates a true anaphylactic reaction but not mediated by immunoglobulins Histamine release Complement activation Direct chemotoxicity (due to electrically charged components) Inhibition of acetylcholinesterase Increased autonomic nervous system activity/patient anxiety
Prevention	Ensure patient well hydrated (>100 mL/h of fluid 4 h before CM and till 24 h post-study) Use of LOCM instead of HOCM Smaller doses Separate two CM studies by at least 48 h Avoid concurrent nephrotoxic drugs for >24 h prior to study Consider use of mannitol or diuretics Consider early hemodialysis in renal failure patients	Use of LOCM can decrease incidence of reactions by 80% Avoid contrast study in patients with previous history of reactions Prophylactic steroids (prednisolone 32 mg orally 12 h and 2 h prior to CM injection) will reduce risk

TABLE 3.2. The European Society of Urogenital Radiology guidelines—Summary

	Renal function	Recommendations
Elective study	Serum creatinine normal	Stop metformin and proceed with study (use LOCM) Check creatinine after 48 h and restart metformin if normal
	Serum creatinine abnormal	Stop metformin for 48 h and then perform study Check creatinine after 48 h and restart metformin if normal
Emergency study	Serum creatinine normal	Stop metformin and proceed with study (use LOCM) Check creatinine after 48 h and restart metformin if normal
	Serum creatinine abnormal	Avoid a contrast study if possible If study essential— Stop metformin Ensure sufficient hydration Proceed with study Monitor serum creatinine, serum lactic acid, serum pH Recommence metformin once creatinine at baseline

(c) ULTRASOUND SCANNING (USS)

Overview
- USS relies on a dual-mode transducer, which first sends high-frequency sound waves into the patient and then receives the reflected waves to generate an image
- Images may be displayed as a two-dimensional gray-scale image or as a color Doppler
- Frequencies used in medical sonography range from 2 to 10 MHz
- The higher the frequency, the better the resolution, but the poorer the depth of penetration. Small part probes for scanning testes and the penis operate at a frequency of between 7 MHz and 9 MHz, while an abdominal scan in an obese individual requires a 2.5–7 MHz transducer

Ultrasound scanning is cheap, easily accessible, painless, safe for the patient, and provides excellent real-time anatomical as well as functional information on the entire urinary tract.

Indications
1. Kidneys, adrenals, and ureter
   - Possible upper tract obstruction (Fig. 3.3a)
   - Suspected renal/adrenal mass (Fig. 3.3b)
   - Investigation of renal failure
   - Investigation of hematuria
   - Monitor renal cystic disease
   - Diagnosis of urinary stone disease
   - Aids access to kidneys for interventional procedures

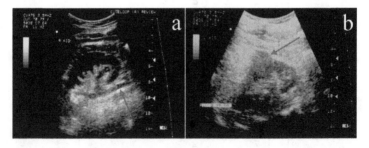

FIGURE 3.3. USS showing (**a**) mild hydronephrosis and dilated upper ureter, (**b**) 4-cm solid RCC interpolar region of kidney (Courtesy of Dr A Bradley, Wythenshawe, Manchester)

- Color doppler to demonstrate vascular lesions
- Visualize a transplanted kidney
- Visualize peri-renal area and the retroperitoneum

2. Bladder
   - Bladder outflow obstruction—measurement of residual urine
   - Investigate intra-vesical mass (e.g., clots, stone, tumor)
   - Aid suprapubic aspiration

3. Prostate and seminal vesical
   - Suspected prostate cancer (+biopsy)
   - Investigation for chronic pelvic pain

4. Scrotum
   - Lump
   - Pain
   - Trauma

5. Penis
   - Investigation of erectile dysfunction
   - Peyronie's disease
   - Diagnose high-flow priapism
   - Can aid visualization of urethral strictures

Technique and radiation

No specific preparation is required for US sonography. It is beyond the scope of this book to describe the vast array of sonographic abnormalities, and therefore only brief principles will be discussed.

- Kidneys and retroperitoneum can be examined in the supine, prone, or decubitus position
- The right kidney is best approached with the patient in a supine position and using the liver as a "viewing window"
- The left kidney is optimally seen with the patient in the right decubitus position with the spleen as an acoustic window
- All other urinary organs, except for the prostate, can be scanned with the patient in the prone position. Trans-rectal USS of the prostate is discussed in a later chapter

The use of color doppler sonography can demonstrate pathologies affecting arterial and venous flow, such as malformations, occlusions, and aneurysms. This is particularly useful in investigation of—

- Kidneys (renal blood flow, renal artery stenosis, renal vein, tumor thrombus). (NB. Fasting for 6–8 hours is helpful for examination of renal arterial flow)

- Scrotal contents (testicular artery blood flow)
- Penile vasculature (cavernosal blood flow)

Finally, USS poses no radiation risk and is the investigation of choice for repeated examinations.

Contrast-enhanced ultrasound

Contrast-enhanced ultrasound (CEUS) is a rapidly expanding field and has been extensively used in the diagnosis and characterization of hepatic lesions. However, due to the inherent vascular nature of the kidneys, CEUS allows excellent spatial and temporal resolution, as well as assessment of renal perfusion.

Contrast agents (SonoVue, Levovist, Optison, Definity, Sonazoid) are intravenously injected compounds which consist of microbubbles containing a gas (air or hydrophobic gas) stabilized by a shell. Thus the agents acting as vascular tracers neither leave the blood vessels nor are subjected to renal filtration, and therefore dramatically increase the signal intensity from blood. Although modern contrast agents are more stable, the microbubble shells are thin and fragile, breaking easily as they oscillate under the influence of the ultrasonic accoustic pressure wave. Even the destruction of the microbubbles can aid in their detection and allow for quantification of renal perfusion. Contrast agents are—

- Safe
- Can be given in a small bolus dose or as a continuous infusion
- Independent of renal function
- Non-nephrotoxic
- Rarely cause allergic reactions

It is likely that given time, CEUS will become more readily available than CT or MR. Disadvantages include the requirement of dedicated contrast-specific software to exploit the many possibilities of CEUS fully and the inability of contrast agents to concentrate in urine, as in IVU and CT. Possible urological applications include—

- Vascular applications
  1. Renal artery stenosis (RAS)—the use of CEUS, rather than doppler will readily demonstrate the entire renal vasculature, including small parenchymal vessels, and has been shown to improve the diagnosis of RAS by enhancing Doppler signals, shortening examination time and decreasing the number of unsuccessful studies

2. Renal vein thrombosis—a small thrombus overlooked by Doppler, may be better demonstrated by CEUS
3. To demonstrate renal blood flow and quantify renal perfusion in the transplanted kidney as well as following suspected renal trauma
4. Parenchymal perfusion—a well perfused parenchyma will exhibit intense contrast-aided enhancement. Therefore CEUS is highly sensitive for the detection of non-perfused lesions including renal cysts, lacerations, infarctions (local underperfusion) and severe pyelonephritis (global underperfusion)

- Focal renal lesions—Small and/or indeterminate focal renal lesions detected by CT or MR are not uncommon in urological practice. CEUS may be superior to conventional USS in the evaluation of such lesions. The absence of any enhancement in a clearly defined cystic lesion would be virtually diagnostic of a benign pathology, due to the lack of blood vessels. Contrast enhancement within renal tumors is often indistinguishable from surrounding parenchyma, but abnormal vascularity frequently seen in tumors is readily identified
- Pediatric—Contrast-enhanced voiding ultrasonography using intravesical Levovist has been demonstrated to have a diagnostic efficacy comparable to standard micturiting cystourethrogram (concordance rate 91%), while avoiding the need for ionizing radiation

Interpretation

1. Kidneys and adrenals

The kidneys must be viewed in both sagittal and transverse planes and a systematic approach is essential.

Size/contour:

- 9–13 cm in length
- Difference of >1.5 cm between the two kidneys is suggestive of a unilateral pathological process

Echogenicity:

- Cortex is homogenous (generally equal or less echoic compared to liver or spleen)
- Thickness of preserved renal cortex usually correlates with renal function
- Central echogenic complex contains the hilar vessels and intrarenal collecting system

- Splaying of the central echogenic complex is seen in hydronephrosis

Masses:

- US is excellent at distinguishing between solid and cystic masses over 2 cm
- Cystic masses are typically spherical with a clearly defined thin wall and demonstrate no internal echoes allowing enhancement of ultrasound transmission. These are generally benign and therefore require no further scrutiny (US diagnostic accuracy virtually 100%)
- Presence of internal echoes, poorly defined walls, and lack of ultrasound transmission is characteristic of a solid mass (USS diagnostic accuracy >84%) and CT evaluation is mandatory

Hydronephrosis:

- Diagnostic accuracy of USS for hydronephrosis is 90–100%
- USS cannot distinguish between obstructive and non-obstructive hydronephrosis
- Other conditions mimicking hydronephrosis include congenital megacalycosis, calyceal diverticulum, parapelvic cysts and prominent extrarenal pelvis
- Conversely, early obstruction, dehydration, and urine extravasation can result in false negatives
- A resistive index (RI) of >0.7 can help distinguish between obstructive and non-obstructive hydronephrosis

RI = max renal artery blood flow (RBF) – min RBF / max RBF

- The extent of dilatation may also be evident (e.g., renal pelvis, ureteric, or bladder)

Vasculature:

- Renal artery stenosis, renal vein thrombosis, and aretriovenous fistulae can easily be demonstrated using color Doppler

Perirenal:

- Urinoma, hematoma, and perinephric abscess can be diagnosed and, in many instances, treated using ultrasound-guided drainage techniques

Retroperitoneum:

• Lymph node enlargement, retroperitoneal tumors, and the aorta can be seen using USS

Adrenal:

• USS visualization is very useful, especially in children
• Small lesions may be missed and a CT scan is advisable in case of persisting doubt

2. Bladder
The bladder can be scanned using the following approaches—

• Transabdominal
• Transrectal
• Transurethral

The transurethral approach provides excellent definition and can be useful in the evaluation of muscle invasion by tumors. The 5.5 MHz transducer (either 90^0 or 135^0) fits within a standard resectoscope. The full bladder should be anechoic and therefore stones, tumors, debris, clots, and infection may cause abnormal echoes.

Bladder urine volume can be measured although inaccurately (volume = height × width × depth/2). Absence of ureteric jets (seen using color Doppler) for >15 min is suggestive of ureteric obstruction. Lower ureteric and vesicoureteric stones can be demonstrated using the transabdominal USS technique.

3. Scrotum
High-frequency, small-parts transducers permit high-quality sonographic evaluation of scrotal contents for abnormal masses (solid and cystic), inflammatory conditions, and blood flow. Doppler flow measurements have a 98% accuracy rate in the diagnosis of acute testicular torsion, but in most cases immediate surgical exploration (rather than USS) is recommended. Doppler studies may also demonstrate high blood flow in the presence of varicoceles and inflammation.

4. Penis
USS of the penis has been used for the following conditions:

1. Impotence: doppler studies can demonstrate cavernosal and internal pudendal blood flow

2. Peyronie's disease: the area of fibrosis or plaque formation is often seen easily using USS
3. Priapism: USS can help differentiate between high-flow (due to arteriovenous fistula) and low-flow priapism
4. Urethral strictures: strictures of the distal urethra and peri-urethral structures can be seen clearly using USS, avoiding the need for unnecessary radiation

5. Intra-operative ultrasound
Intra-operative ultrasound (IUSS) allows visualization of tissues without distortion by abdominal organs, bowel gas, and bony structures and will be used increasingly in the future. Applications for renal surgery include assessment of—

- Whether a tumor is amenable for partial nephrectomy by delineating tumor anatomy
- Local vasculature using color Doppler
- Renal vein involvement by tumor
- Use of real-time laparoscopic IUSS for laparoscopic renal cryo-surgery and high-intensity focused ultrasound (HIFU)

Advantages
- Safe—no radiation involved
- Non-invasive
- Cheap—therefore readily available
- No requirement for intravenous contrast
- Not dependent on function
- Excellent anatomical detail
- Occasional functional/physiological information
- Doppler studies excellent for vascular/flow studies
- Useful adjunct to interventional procedures (e.g., nephros-tomy, abscess drainage)

Drawbacks
- Operator dependent
- Equipment dependent (more expensive machines provide better resolution)
- Limited by patient's body habitus—presence of intervening fat, bowel gas, bony structures, surgical wounds, and dressings can compromise image quality
- Image quality can be inferior compared to IVU and CT scanning
- Offers little functional information

- Retroperitoneal structures, including ureters, may not be seen easily

---

(d) COMPUTED TOMOGRAPHY (CT)

Introduction
The advances in computed tomography (CT) scanning have revolutionized uroradiological imaging, such that in many practices it often is the first—and only—investigation performed for a variety of urological complaints. Collimation allows a rotating thin beam of X-rays to pass through the patient's body, which is attenuated by absorption and scattered as it is passed through the patient. A computer produces a composite image using the transmitted beams.

The present third- and fourth-generation CT scanners are faster and offer outstanding picture definition. The current spiral (helical) CT scanners permit continuous X-ray exposure through a fast rotating X-ray tube (often one rotation in <1 s), thereby allowing superior images for 3D reconstruction. CT scanning technology continues to develop, and it is beyond the realm of this book to deal with the entire array of radiological techniques and findings. Therefore only important principles pertaining to urological practice are highlighted.

Indications
1. Kidneys
   - Detection, definition, and staging of renal masses (Fig. 3.4a–c)
   - Delineation of complex renal stones
   - Evaluation of renal vasculature (e.g., renal artery stenosis, aneurysms, a-v malformations, aberrant crossing lower pole vessels)
   - Characterization of perirenal and bladder inflammatory masses (Fig. 3.4d)
   - Investigation of level and cause of hydronephrosis
   - Investigation of filling defects in the collecting system (Fig. 3.4e)
   - Extent and staging of renal tract trauma
   - Evaluation of renal transplants
   - Investigation of congenital renal malformations
   - Adjunct to interventional procedures (e.g., renal biopsy, puncture)

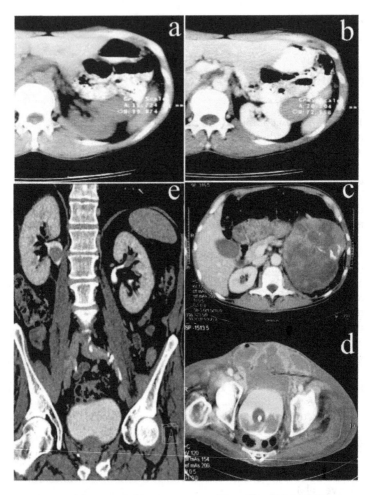

FIGURE 3.4. (**a**) Pre- and (**b**) post-contrast CT papillary RCC left kidney—mass enhances from 40 to 72 HU, (**c**) large left RCC, (**d**) CT pelvis showing abscess cavity anterior to the bladder secondary to a bladder perforation, (**e**) bilateral upper tract TCC (Courtesy of Dr A Bradley, Wythenshawe, Manchester)

2. Retroperitoneum
   • CT scanning is the investigation of choice for the assessment of retroperitoneal lymph nodes, masses, abscess or fibrosis

3. Ureter
   • Suspected ureteric stones (accuracy >97% with non-contrast CT scan) (Fig. 3.5)
4. Adrenal
   • Investigation of suspected adrenal mass
5. Bladder
   • Staging of invasive bladder tumors
6. Prostate and seminal vesicals
   • Staging of prostate tumors
   • Investigation of abscess, congenital deformities, and cysts
7. Testes
   • Detection of metastases from testis cancer

Technique and radiation

Contrast
Oral contrast will opacify bowel and avoid confusion of fluid-filled bowel and abdominal masses and lymph nodes. Water-soluble contrast medium (20 mL of Urografin 150 diluted with 1 L of orange squash) or low-density barium suspensions (2% w/v) can be used. Further details are given in Table 3.3. Oral contrast is not required when performing CT angiography or unenhanced CT for detection of renal calculi.

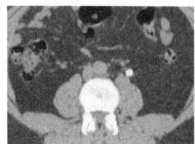
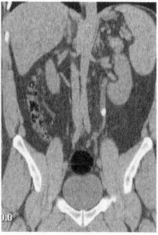

FIGURE 3.5. Non-contrast CT showing left ureteric stone in (**a**) axial and (**b**) coronal views (Courtesy of Dr A Bradley, Wythenshawe, Manchester)

TABLE 3.3. Oral contrast for CT

	Contrast Volume (mL)	Time Before Scan
Adult		
Abdomen and pelvis	1,000	Gradually over 1 h before scan
Renal only	500	Gradually over 30 min before scan
Child		
Newborn	60–90	
1 mo–1 yr	120–240	Full dose 1 h before scan and a further half-dose immediately prior to scan
1 yr–10 yr	240–480	
>10 yr	Adult dose	
If colon needs to be opacified, then give contrast night before scan		

Intravenous (IV) contrast should be given in virtually all urological patients, except when looking for a renal tract calculi. Intravenous contrast permits—

- Improved delineation of renal masses
- Evaluation of surrounding vasculature
- Characterization of masses by their pattern of contrast enhancement. The contraindications and side effects of intravenous contrast agents have been discussed earlier (see Chapter 3b: IVU)

The standard renal mass protocol is based on renal enhancement post IV contrast injection.

1. Non-contrast scan: best for identification of renal tract calculi, fat, and baseline enhancement
2. Arterial (cortical) phase scan: 15–25 seconds after contrast injection allows evaluation of renal arteries
3. Corticomedullary (nephrographic) phase scan: 70–120 seconds after contrast injection allows visualization of renal parenchymal anatomy. Also provides good hepatic and portal vein enhancement

4. Excretory phase scan: 3–5 min after contrast injection allows evaluation of the collecting system and renal pelvis

Delaying the scan beyond this period will demonstrate opacification of the ureters and bladder.

Enhancement (Hounsfield units)
Tissue enhancement (density/attenuation value) is standardized on the Hounsfield scale. The scale extends from −1,000 to +1,000 Hounsfield units (HU) (see Table 3.4). Enhancement of >10 HU post-contrast compared to the non-contrast phase is indicative of a solid, enhancing, malignant mass.

Data processing and images
3D reconstruction—With the increased use of multislice CT scanners, it is now possible to obtain a large number of very thin (<2.5 mm) cross-sectional axial images of the entire urinary tract in a matter of minutes. In addition, these images can be displayed in a variety of multiplanar and 3D reformatted images. Currently, one of three different 3D reconstructions algorithms may be used:

- Average-intensity projection (most closely resembles IVU images)
- Maximum-intensity projection
- Volume rendering

Evidence of the superiority of one over the other is not available yet, but volume rendering seems to be the most preferred owing to the fact that image creation is quick, is least dependent on

TABLE 3.4. Hounsfield scale

Tissue	Hounsfield Units (HU)
Bone	+1,000
Renal tract calculus	>+400
Non-specific calcification	>+150
Acute hemorrhage	+50 to 90
Clotted blood	+70
Soft tissue	+10 to +50
Water	0
Fat	−50 to −100
Air	−1,000

technical factors, and provides excellent data-rich images of the urinary tract in its entirety without any loss of information. The improved resolution and accuracy of reconstructed images, combined with CT angiography, is increasing its use in a range of conditions where demonstration of renal and perirenal vasculature is essential, including—

- Assessment and staging of renal tumors
- Planning for nephron-sparing surgery
- Prior to surgery for uretero-pelvic junction obstruction surgery (e.g., endopyelotomy)
- Prior to complex stone surgery
- Assessment of renal transplant donors
- Arterio-venous malformation
- Assessment of complex urinary fistulas

It is important to study the actual axial 2D images as certain small lesions may not be easily identified on reconstructed images. In one recent study, standard 2D CT images correctly demonstrated 89% of small upper tract TCC, compared to a 25% pick-up rate with 3D reconstruction images.

Virtual endoscopy
By using a surface-rendering technique, CT images can be utilized to enable imaging of hollow organs such as the bladder and ureter. Virtual endoscopy—

- Has the main advantage of being non-invasive
- Permits good visualization of the tumor morphology as well as reasonable demonstration of the bladder/ureter wall
- Is unable to detect flat mucosal lesions, such as carcinoma in situ
- Imparts no data with regard to tumor grade and stage

The overall sensitivity and specificity of virtual ureteroscopy are 81% and 100%, respectively, for the detection of polypoidal ureteric lesions, and 80% and 75% for the detection of upper tract TCC. While virtual cystoscopy is unlikely ever to gain popularity in the assessment of bladder cancers, virtual ureteroscopy may, with further refinements, be incorporated into the management of selected patient groups (e.g., patients unfit for repeated general anesthetic procedures, single kidneys, surveillance in patients with previous upper tract TCC).

The effective radiation dose for a non-contrast abdominal CT scan is 8 mSv (equivalent to 4 years of background radiation or 20,000 miles traveled by car). However, performing a four-phase contrast CT urography can expose the patient to an effective radiation dose of 25–35 mSv (at least five times that of the IVU).

Interpretation

1. Kidneys and surrounding structures

The kidneys are easily seen in the retroperitoneum within Gerota's fascia, with surrounding perinephric fat. A careful and systematic examination is made of the kidneys, renal vessels, collecting system, peri-renal tissue, adrenals and the rest of the retroperitoneum. Basis principles are discussed below.

- Renal cysts
  - Most common of all renal masses
  - USS usually able to distinguish between solid and cystic masses
  - Doubt may exist with 20–40% of renal lesions
  - CT scan alone has an accuracy approaching 100%
  - For a simple renal cyst to be considered thus, all of the following stringent criteria must be met:
    a. Homogenous water density contents with attenuation no greater than 20 HU
    b. Smooth-contoured, rounded, or oval shape without a perceptible wall
    c. No contrast enhancement

Any other cysts must be considered complex and further enquiry is mandatory. Bosniak has proposed the following categorization of cystic renal masses based on CT findings:

- Category I: (benign) simple benign cyst meeting all the CT criteria described above
- Category II: (usually benign, but 13–27% malignant) simple cystic lesions which are minimally complicated including septation; minimal calcification; obviously infected and non-enhancing high-density cysts (category IIF—these cysts are more complex and cannot be neatly categorized into type II or III. These may contain a slightly increased number of hairline septa; minimal but smooth thickening of septa wall; contain

calcification. The "F" indicates the need for follow-up imaging)

- Category III: (between 45% and 60% malignant) more complicated cysts which demonstrate findings associated with malignancy including multi-loculation; hemorrhage; coarse calcification; non-enhancing solid components
- Category IV: (about 90% malignant) clearly malignant lesions with cystic components; irregular and enhancing solid areas

Thin areas of linear calcification within cyst walls, or thin septations within a cyst are of no significance when noted in isolation. High-density areas, calcification, and hemorrhage noted in patients with polycystic kidney disease can often mimic malignant changes.

- Renal cell carcinoma (RCC)

  - Typically appears as solid masses
  - Frequently associated with hemorrhage, necrosis, and calcification
  - Pre-contrast attenuation is similar to that of the surrounding renal parenchyma (+30 to +60 HU), with obvious enhancement following contrast injection (but to a lesser degree than the parenchyma)
  - Allows accurate staging of RCC and provides information on—
    ◊ Tumor size
    ◊ Local invasion
    ◊ Venous involvement
    ◊ Tumor vascularity (using angiography techniques)
    ◊ Presence of obvious lymph node metastases

- Renal lymphoma

One in 20 of all patients with lymphoma will have renal involvement, and separating these lesions from metastatic renal deposits (from an extra-renal source) can prove challenging. Retroperitoneal lymphadenopathy is almost always observed with renal lymphoma. CT scanning may reveal single or multiple, unilateral or bilateral, enhancing parenchymnal lesion, or may demonstrate diffuse renal infiltrative enlargement.

- Upper tract TCC

  - CT has a poorly defined role in the management of upper tract urothelial malignancies

- Reported sensitivities have been as high as 89–98% (compared to between 60% and 79% for retrograde pyelograms) but false-negative rates are disappointing
- Unlikely to replace direct access endoscopic visualization of the renal tract
- Ureteric or renal pelvic TCC may appear as either filling defects, mass lesions, or urothelial thickening
- Main role is in the detection of lymph node or extra-urinary metastases

- Angiomyolipoma

  - Benign lesions
  - May be confused with RCC
  - Characterized by their gross fat content
  - Diagnosis must be suspected in the pre-contrast films (by the presence of fat) as post-contrast enhancement usually occurs due to the vascular nature of these lesions
  - Angiomyolipomas contain both muscle and vascular elements and appear as large, low-density, irregular, fatty tumors, and may be associated with surrounding hemorrhage
  - Bilateral lesions are usually associated with tuberous sclerosis

- Oncocytoma

  - Renal oncocytomas often difficult to diagnose pre-operatively
  - CT angiography may demonstrate a large, homogenous, well-circumscribed central mass with a scar, surrounded by a "spoke-wheel" configuration of tumor vessels
  - Confusion with an RCC is common

- Hydronephrosis

  - CT scanning has a false-negative rate of 10–20% for the detection of hydronephrosis
  - May provide useful information of the degree and level of obstruction as well as preservation of renal cortex
  - Contrast extravasation is a feature of acute obstruction
  - Mild hydronephrosis—minor splaying of renal fat and sinus structures secondary to pelvi-calyceal dilatation
  - Moderate hydronephrosis—more prominent dilatation of the collecting system
  - Severe hydronephrosis—marked dilatation with minimal or no contrast, in association with loss of cortex

- Renal calculi

    - Non-contrast CT has a detection rate approaching 100% for all types of renal calculi
    - Calcium and oxalate containing stones have an attenuation value of between +400 and +1,200 HU
    - Less dense cystine and uric acid stones measure in at between +100 to +200 HU

- Inflammatory lesions

    - USS may be sufficient in the majority of patients with inflammatory conditions affecting the kidneys
    - CT gives superior imaging compared to USS and IVU
    - CT indicated in patients unresponsive to antimicrobial therapy
    - Acute pyelonephritis may reveal a diffusely enlarged kidney with general or focal wedge-shaped areas of diminished contrast enhancement
    - Renal and perirenal abscesses containing pus, stones, blood, and gas are easily visible
    - Xanthogranulomatous pyelonephritis, seen in patients with a history of chronic infection, is usually secondary to stone disease and is frequently characterized by the presence of renal calculi within a fibrotic kidney containing multiple abscess cavities

- Renal trauma

CT is the investigation of choice in the initial assessment of the extent of renal trauma. The advantages of CT include (i) reasonably quick examination, (ii) non-invasive, (iii) contrast use allows for good demonstration of even subtle arterial or venous injuries, (iv) can identify non-renal organ injuries.

Indications for CT imaging following renal trauma include—

   i. Penetrating trauma
  ii. Clinical suspicion of other abdominal or retroperitoneal organ injury
 iii. Blunt trauma, if associated with macroscopic hematuria
  iv. Blunt trauma with microscopic hematuria, plus either (1) shock (systolic BP <90 mmHg at any time) or (2) clinical suspicion of additional abdominal organ injury, or (3) significant deceleration injury (e.g., fall from height)

Using helical CT, a two-phase technique is recommended. Immediate films following contrast injection will permit diagnosis of reno-vascular injury, while a delayed (5–20 min) scan will aid recognition of injury to the collecting system or ureters.

Renal pedical injuries are accurately diagnosed with CT. Complete renal artery or segmental arterial occlusions are seen as absence of contrast enhancement in whole or part of the kidney. Complete renal artery occlusion usually results in an absent nephrogram, but may also demonstrate the "rim sign" (peripheral cortical enhancement due to collateral arterial supply).

The severity of renal trauma can be accurately assessed and graded using the American Association for the Surgery of Trauma system (Table 3.5).

- Adrenals

  - Primary radiological investigation for suspected adrenal masses
  - Virtually all masses >1 cm diameter are easily identified
  - Lipomas and adenomas have a higher lipid content and low enhancement (<10 HU)
  - CT will readily distinguish between cysts and malignant masses

TABLE 3.5. American Association for the Surgery of Trauma Classification for renal trauma

Grade	Type	Description
1	Contusion	Subcapsular injury with no parenchymal lacerations
2	Hematoma	Renal laceration (limited to cortex or <1 cm parenchymal depth); non-expanding peri-renal hematoma confined to retroperitoneum; no urine extravasation (*75–85% of renal traumas are ≤grade 2*)
3	Deep laceration	Deep laceration involving medulla (depth >1 cm) not involving collecting system; no urine extravasation; segmental arterial thrombosis
4	Deep laceration	Laceration extending through cortex, medulla, and collecting system; urinary extravasation; main renal artery or vein injury with contained hemorrhage
5	Laceration/ vascular	Shattered kidney; renal pedicle avulsion (causing devascularisation of kidney); renal artery thrombosis

(add one grade for bilateral injuries up to grade 3)

- Distinguishing between an adrenal adenoma and adrenal metastases can prove more difficult
- Bilateral adrenal masses are more suggestive of secondaries or lymphoma
- Masses >2 cm are likely to be malignant

2. CT of the pelvis

Traditionally, CT scanning has been the primary imaging modality in the staging of bladder and prostate cancer, but recent evidence suggests that magnetic resonance imaging (MRI) provides superior resolution and therefore may be more accurate. In addition, metastatic disease within the pelvis is easily demonstrated on CT.

On CT, normal lymph nodes are up to 10 mm in maximum transverse diameter in the para-aortic and iliac chains, and 6 mm in the retrocrural region. While this size criteria is reasonably accurate, CT cannot differentiate between lymphadenopathy secondary to tumor or inflammation. It is also well recognized that tumor infiltration may be present in smaller nodes considered insignificant on the basis of size criteria.

- Bladder cancer

  - Bladder tumors may be seen as mass lesions, filling defects, or bladder wall thickenings on CT
  - CT is reasonably accurate (70–88%) at detecting locally advanced tumor (stage T3b and above)
  - CT is unable to distinguish between tumors of a lower stage and over-staging is a distinct possibility
  - Accuracy of CT for lymph node detection lies between 70% and 92%
  - CT is primarily utilized for patients with advanced disease or those at risk of metastatic spread

- Prostate cancer

  - MRI scanning is now the principal imaging technique for CAP
  - CT cannot distinguish between the various grades of organ-confined disease
  - CT able to detect local invasion into bladder or seminal vesicals and the presence of gross lymphadenopathy
  - overall accuracy of CT in the staging of prostate cancer varies between 50% and 80%
  - CT unable to differentiate confidently between malignant and benign conditions involving the prostate

- Bladder trauma

As an alternative to conventional retrograde contrast cystogram in patients with suspected bladder trauma, up to 400 mL of diluted iodinated contrast (4%) can be inserted into the bladder via a urethral or suprapubic catheter prior to performing a CT scan (CT cystography). Bladder rupture may be intra- (involving the dome of bladder) or extra-peritoneal.

Overall advantages and disadvantages

Advantages

- Single imaging technique for visualization of the entire renal tract with excellent anatomical detail
- Simultaneously detects non-urological pathology (e.g., liver)
- Identifies virtually all renal and ureteric calculi
- Increased sensitivity in detection of renal masses
- Allows accurate staging of detected malignancies
- 3D reconstruction enables delineation of anatomy and aids surgical planning
- CT angiography (non-invasive) as accurate as conventional angiography (invasive)

Drawbacks

- Radiation risk to patient
- Often requires intravenous contrast with its associated risks
- Limitations in stone disease—oral contrast may be excreted in urine and conceal small stones; obstruction secondary to calculus may not be apparent (whereas obstruction is usually obvious with conventional IVU)
- Expensive (and therefore limited availability of scanners and technology for analysis)
- Large variety of techniques with no clear consensus for best technique
- Interpretation requires time and expertise
- Prone to technical artifacts—due to patient movement or partial volume averaging of adjacent organs
- Poor accuracy for luminal pathology (and therefore inadequate for staging of low-stage pelvic disease)

(e) MAGNETIC RESONANCE IMAGING (MRI)

Overview

Recent years have seen an increase in the usage of magnetic resonance imaging (MRI) to image the urinary tract. Faster scanners can now provide high-resolution multiplanar images for accurate diagnosis. While it is beyond the scope of this book to elucidate the physics of MRI, an understanding of basic principles is desirable. The fundamental basis of MR scanning is the conversion of radiofrequency energy into gray scale, to allow production of an image.

Nuclei, with unpaired electrons, behave like tiny magnets. The hydrogen nuclei (proton), ubiquitously found throughout the human body in water and body fat, align themselves when placed within an external magnetic field. The magnetic fields used in clinical practice are potent and range from 0.15–1.5 tesla (1,500 to 15,000 gauss) as compared with the earth's magnetic field of 0.5 gauss. This alignment of protons forms the basis of the MR signal. A radiofrequency pulse applied to the protons will cause the protons to absorb energy and deviate from alignment with the external magnetic field. Withdrawal of the radiofrequency pulse will therefore allow relaxation of the protons (i.e., protons realign with the magnetic field) to their resting state. The return of the proton to alignment with the magnetic field is termed T_1 relaxation. In addition, relaxation of the protons back to their resting state also results in a redistribution of the protons, such that two protons starting out next to each other will end up separated with time. This process is termed T_2 relaxation.

Thus a T_1-weighted scan is mainly (but not exclusively) due to the effects of T_1 relaxation and shows better anatomical detail and better separation of solid and cystic masses. A T_2-weighted scan is mostly influenced by T_2 relaxation and is more sensitive in detecting local pathology (tumors, hematomas, inflammation). Although each tissue has its characteristic properties with regard to T_1 and T_2, MR images can be changed and manipulated to highlight different aspects of the organ/lesion being studied. In contrast to axial CT pictures, MR images can readily be produced in any other plane, including sagittal and coronal. MR images can be used to produce angiogram-like images of the vasculature of any organ, and thus magnetic resonance angiography (MRA) is an effective, non-invasive alternative to conventional angiography. MR does not utilize ionizing radiation, which is an inherent advantage.

Indications
1. Kidneys
   - Assessment of indeterminate renal masses (MR will readily distinguish between cysts and other benign or malignant neoplasms)
   - Staging of renal cell carcinoma

- Renal lymphoma (CT often is insufficient for the detection of renal involvement)
- MRA allows excellent demonstration of renal vasculature and is useful if suspicion of renal artery stenosis, renal vein occlusion, renal artery aneurysms, and arteriovenous malformations
- Retroperitoneal fibrosis (may help distinguish between a malignant or benign etiology)
- Assessment of the transplanted kidney
- MR urography can be performed to assess for calculi or obstruction if conventional iodinated contrast techniques are contraindicated (e.g., pregnancy, renal failure) (Fig. 3.6b)

2. Adrenal
   - Pheochromocytoma
   - To distinguish between adrenal adenoma, carcinoma, and metastases
3. Bladder
   - Staging of bladder tumor (Fig. 3.6a)
4. Prostate
   - Staging of prostate cancer (Fig. 3.6c,d)
5. Penis and testis
   - No absolute indication, but MR can be used in the examination of a variety of benign (including detection of the undescended testis) and malignant disease processes

Technique and radiation

No specific preparation is required for patients undergoing MR scanning. It is however important to be aware of certain important contraindications:

- Pacemakers, cochlear implants, implanted infusion pumps, and other implanted devices can malfunction in the strong magnetic field
- Cerebral aneurysm clips, older (Bjork–Shiley) heart valves, titanium intravascular filters, metallic foreign objects (e.g., bullets, shrapnel, fragments in the eye) may undergo deflection
- Patients with claustrophobia, patients with dementia (who may be unable to remain still in the scanner), and morbidly obese patients (due to limited gantry space) are unsuitable

Most modern orthopedic implants are safe. Patients must be warned about possible noise levels, which may reach up 95 dB on occasions. In spite of the lack of evidence linking MR to

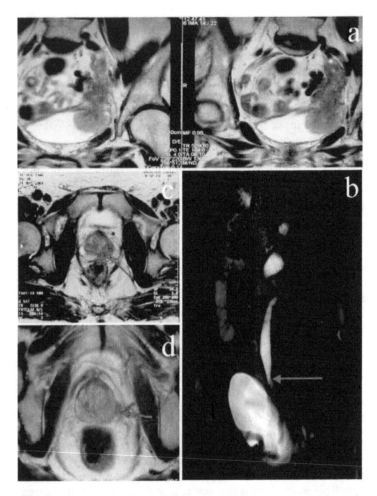

FIGURE 3.6. (a) T2-weighted MRI showing left lower ureteric TCC invading the bladder, (b) sagittal T2 MR urogram in an 18-week pregnant female showing ureter narrowing where it crosses the iliac vessels (c) and (d) axial T2 MR prostate—low signal tumor replacing the normal high signal PZ on the left, with early extracapsular disease on the left (Courtesy of Dr A Bradley, Wythenshawe, Manchester)

teratogenesis, MR scanning is not advised in pregnancy, especially in the first trimester. Nevertheless, in later pregnancy, MR urography may be utilised in the investigation of suspected upper tract obstruction (e.g., secondary to a ureteric calculus).

In order to enhance the inherent contrast between tissues, contrast agents, such as gadolinium chelate, may be used.

Gadolinium—

- Is a paramagnetic metal
- Shortens the T_1 relaxation time
- Is freely filtered and excreted by the kidneys
- Is non-nephrotoxic
- Is rarely associated with allergic reactions
- Can be used safely in patients with compromised renal function, except in severe renal impairment (GFR <20 mL/min), in which case MR scanning must be followed up by dialysis

Some of the signal intensities of commonly encountered urological tissues are given in Table 3.6.

TABLE 3.6. Signal intensities of urological tissues

Substance	T_1 Weighted	T_2 Weighted
Kidneys		
Cortex/medulla	Gray (medium intensity)	White (high intensity)
Urine (water)	Black (low intensity)	White
Renal cell carcinoma	Gray	White/gray
Simple cyst	Black	White
Hemorrhagic cyst	White	White
Bladder—detrussor muscle	Black	Black
Prostate/seminal vesicles		
Peripheral zone	Gray-white	White
Transitional zone	Gray	Black
Prostate cancer	Gray	Gray-white
Seminal vesicles	Black	White
Adrenal	Gray	Gray
Cyst	Black	White
Pheochromocytoma	Gray	Bright white
Blood flow—fast	Black	Black
Tumor thrombus	Gray	Gray
Lymph nodes	Gray	Gray
Fat	White	Gray-white
Bone	Black	Black
Marrow	Bright white	White
Metastases	Gray	Black

There is no ionizing radiation risk to patients undergoing MR, hence it is useful in pregnant women (Fig. 3.6b). A number of potential hazards have been reported, including effects of magnetic fields (minor alterations in the electrocardiogram, length of the cardiac cycle, RBC morphology, and nerve excitability); visual flashes (due to optic pathway stimulation); and burns (conduction loops) or frostbite (coolant gases). Nevertheless, these rare events are usually minor and easily reversible on terminating the scan.

Interpretation

1. The kidney and surrounding structures

MR scanning, in contrast to CT, does not require ionizing radiation, utilizes non-nephrotoxic contrast, and will produce better contrast resolution in soft tissues, but is more expensive, less readily available, and therefore only plays a secondary, supportive role in the investigation of kidney diseases.

- Renal masses

  - Renal lesions which remain ambiguous (e.g., hemorrhagic cyst) following CT and USS, can be clarified using MR
  - Cysts do not demonstrate contrast enhancement (T_1 weighted), in contrast to solid lesions
  - Better detection of angiopyolipoma and renal lymphoma compared to CT
  - Accuracy of renal cancer staging by MR is between 70% and 80%
  - Evaluation of venous involvement is correctly demonstrated in 90% to 100% of cases

- Renal vasculature

  - MRA provides a useful, non-invasive technique for the assessment of renal vasculature
  - Can detect renal artery stenosis in transplant, as well as non-transplant patients
  - Avoids use of potentially nephrotoxic contrast media

- MR urography

  - Gadolinium-enhanced MR scanning can satisfactorily map the whole of the collecting system and ureter if scenarios where intravenous contrast is contraindicated (e.g., pregnancy, in children and patients with a history of contrast allergy)

- A small degree of diuresis (e.g., following administration of furosemide) can enhance image quality in the detection of urothelial neoplasms and ureteric obstruction

- Adrenal

  - MR at least as accurate as CT in the detection/characterization of adrenal masses
  - Particularly useful in distinguishing between adenomas and adrenal metastases
  - Can confirm the presence of pheochromocytoma (both adrenal and ectopic)

2. MR of the pelvis

Bladder

Manipulation of MR technique will allow reasonable demonstration of all the layers of the bladder wall, but still remains inferior to direct cystoscopy in the diagnosis of bladder tumors. Intravenous gadolinium produces intense detrussor enhancement. MR (T_2-weighted images) will detect muscle-invasive or locally advanced bladder carcinoma with an accuracy of >90% and has become the standard tool for investigation of invasive bladder cancer prior to radical surgery or radiotherapy. In addition, lower ureteric tumors, tumor within diverticula, and urachal tumors are best demonstrated by MR. Ideally, MR must be deferred for at least 6 weeks following endoscopic resection or biopsy. Artifactual overstaging due to post-resection edema remains a distinct possibility, and all attempts must be made to obtain an MR prior to resection. In addition, non-specific scarring due to post-radiation or peri-vesical inflammation can be confused with malignant extension, resulting in tumor over-staging.

Prostate

In contrast to the bladder, under-staging is seen more often in patients undergoing MR for prostatic adenocarcinoma. MR, especially with an endorectal surface coil, is being extensively utilized to stage prostate cancer locally. T_2-weighted images with an endorectal surface coil will provide excellent visualization of the prostatic zones, capsule, and neurovascular bundles. Pelvic lymphadenopathy is best demonstrated on T_1-weighted body coil images. Although many studies have claimed a sensitivity of >90% for the identification of extracapsular disease, the overall accuracy of MR for the prostatic adenocarcinoma lies between

51% and 82%. MR must be deferred for at least 4 weeks in patients following transrectal biopsy or transurethral prostate resection.

Size criteria for lymph nodes is the same as for CT, although MR is more likely to demonstrate smaller nodes.

3. MR of the external genitalia

Penis
MR can be employed to delineate penile anatomy and is a useful tool in the management of Peyronie's disease (for plaque demonstration), penile fractures, and erectile dysfunction (indications not clearly defined).

Testis
Although MR will readily distinguish between testicular torsion, inflammation, and tumors, the combined high diagnostic accuracy of USS and clinical examination almost negates its routine use in urological practice. MR can however, be utilized in non-emergency cases where doubt exists, as anatomical demonstration is superior with MR compared to USS.

Advantages
- Can image in any plane
- Non-ionizing and therefore perceived to be safe
- Excellent anatomical detail, especially of soft tissue
- Semi-quantitative assessment of perfusion
- Non-invasive angiography (MRA)
- No bony artifact due to lack of signal from bone
- Contrast use is infrequent and safe

Drawbacks
- High operating costs
- Limited availability for emergencies
- Can be slow—although modern scanners are much quicker
- Interpretation requires expertise
- Artifacts may be produced by patient movement
- Artifacts may also be produced due to scarring and inflammation
- Inability to show renal tract calcification
- Tendency to over-stage prostate and bladder cancers
- Fresh hemorrhage not as well visualized as by CT
- Contraindicated in certain patients
- Can be noisy and claustrophobic

(f) MAGNETIC RESONANCE SPECTROSCOPY

Overview

- MRI has a developing role in the management of CAP
- Magnetic resonance spectroscopic imaging (MRSI) combines magnetic resonance and spectroscopy to generate three-dimensional anatomical information with superimposed metabolic data, thus increasing its clinical utility
- MRSI has been tested in renal cancers but most studies have focused on its role in CAP

Alignment of the hydrogen nuclei (proton) within a strong external magnetic field is the basis of MR scanning. Fundamental to MRSI is the observation that signals derived from protons of different molecules differ slightly in their frequencies. A spectral map of signal intensity versus frequency (therefore a spectrum) can then be traced for all the relevant endogenous chemicals (metabolites) which exist in the prostate. The metabolites relevant to the prostate include citrate, choline, creatine, and polyamines which resonate at different frequencies in the spectrum, resulting in signature "peaks" on the spectral trace based on their relative concentrations. Changes in the concentrations of these metabolites are the basis of cancer detection.

At present, despite evidence confirming the superiority of MRSI in the detection and staging of prostate cancer, since it provides functional data which can be combined with structural information (from MRI) resulting in a detailed evaluation of the prostate and pelvis, it remains confined to a few centers and further studies are required to unravel its role in the future.

Indications

The technology and clinical evidence surrounding MRSI continues to evolve, but possible indications include—

- Local staging and detection of capsular involvement
- One or more negative prostate biopsies and a rising PSA; MRSI may assist in directing biopsies
- Detect local recurrence or residual tumor
- Help discriminate whether post-treatment pelvic mass is benign or malignant
- Can aid treatment planning by improving cancer localization prior to external beam radiotherapy or brachytherapy
- Monitor/predict tumor response

Technique and radiation

MRI and MRSI are acquired in the same examination, requiring around 60 minutes. Although no specific patient preparation is required for MRSI, the same exclusion criteria apply as for patients undergoing MRI scanning. For best spectroscopy performance, use of an endorectal coil combined with four external coils is recommended.

Each spectrum is derived from a voxel. A voxel is a small (0.24–$0.34\,cm^3$) volume of prostate, and MRSI produces arrays of contiguous voxels to map the whole prostate. Concentration of the resonating prostatic metabolites are recorded as peaks and the distribution patterns can help distinguish between benign and malignant prostatic tissue. Using specialized software, regions mapped by MRSI are then overlaid on the MRI images to allow correlation of areas of metabolic and anatomical abnormalities.

MRSI appears to be inherently safe and does not involve irradiation of the patient.

Interpretation

A brief summary of recognized biochemical changes within the prostate gland is provided here.

- MRSI in a normal healthy prostate will demonstrate high quantities of citrate, zinc, and polyamines (Fig 3.7A)
- Creatine levels in the prostate appear relatively constant irrespective of the underlying pathological process, and since the spectral peaks of both creatine and choline often overlap, they are often analyzed in combination.
- In CAP—
  - Choline levels increase and citrate levels decrease compared to those found in benign disease (Fig 3.7B)
  - There appears to be a reduction in the concentration of polyamines, although there have been contradictory reports
  - There seems to be a relationship between tumor grade and the choline (+creatine) to citrate ratio, with the magnitude of choline elevation being the most significant predictor of the Gleason score

Some areas of possible clinical application are described below:

- The role of MRSI in the diagnosis of prostate cancer has not been clarified because most patients will only undergo MR imaging after biopsy-proven prostate cancer

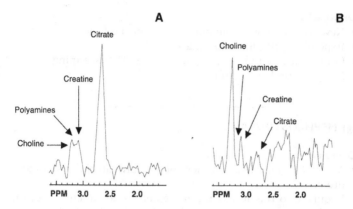

FIGURE 3.7. MR spectroscopy—MR spectral trace from (**A**) normal peripheral zone prostate tissue and (**B**) Gleason 7 peripheral zone prostate cancer (With permission from Elsevier—Coakley, *J Urology*, Vol 170, S69–76, 2003, 170)

- There is emerging evidence that, in patients with an abnormal PSA and negative prostate biopsies, MRSI can aid localization and increase the positive yield of subsequent biopsies
- MRSI is superior to standard MRI in the estimation of tumor volume and detection of capsular/extracapsular involvement (detection rate up to 83%) thereby influencing treatment options. Its main role may well be confined initially to the grading of prostate tumors
- MRSI localization techniques have been used to increase radiation dosage (brachytherapy or external beam) to areas of the prostate with alleged carcinoma
- In treatment failures, MRSI can detect residual tumor following failed radiotherapy and androgen deprivation therapy (detection less favorable following radical prostatectomy). It may also help discriminate between residual/recurrent tumor and benign necrotic/fibrotic tissue following cryosurgery
- Certain cancers may be characterized as high-grade based on spectroscopic patterns and may subsequently respond poorly to treatment

Advantages
- Combination with MR scanning allows simultaneous anatomical and metabolic assessment
- Reasonably high specificity
- Does not involve ionizing radiation
- Non-invasive

Drawbacks
- New technique with incompletely defined efficacy
- Expensive with limited availability
- Contraindicated in certain patients (see MRI scanning)
- Movement-related artifacts

(g) NEPHROSTOGRAM

Overview
- A useful tool in the assessment of the pelvicalyceal system and ureters
- Requisite to this test is the placement of a catheter or drain in the upper urinary tract providing access for contrast delivery
- The collecting system and ureter can be filled with contrast media and fluoroscopy used to acquire the relevant anatomical information

Indications
It is uncommon for a nephrostomy to be inserted simply for purposes of performing a nephrostogram. The more likely clinical scenario is that renal puncture has already been performed for other indications, and a nephrostogram obtained while it remains in position. Indications for a nephrostogram include—

- Assessment of an obstructing lesion (e.g., calculus, tumor, ureteric strictures or UPJ obstruction) when other radiographic modalities have been insufficient (Fig. 3.8a)
- Assess residual stone fragments following percutaneous stone surgery
- Assess response to treatment (e.g., after BCG/mitomycin therapy for ureteric tumor)
- Delineation of ureteric fistulas

Other general indications for nephrostomy insertion also include—

- Drainage of pyonephrosis
- Relief of ureteric obstruction
- Prior to percutaneous nephrolithotomy (PCNL)
- For antegrade ureteric stenting (Fig. 3.8b)
- Performance of perfusion pressure test (Whitaker's test)

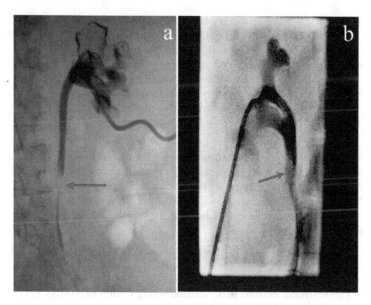

FIGURE 3.8. Nephrostogram—(**a**) radiolucent calculi in the upper pole and proximal ureter, (**b**) nephrostogram and antegrade ureteric stent insertion with obstructing proximal ureteric stone (Courtesy of Dr A Bradley, Wythenshawe, Manchester)

Technique and radiation

Contraindications to renal puncture and performance of nephrostogram include—

1. History of previous allergic reaction to contrast media
2. Bleeding diathesis
3. Presence of urinary sepsis (when puncture is mandatory, i.e., for drainage of pyonephrosis, prophylactic and post-procedure antibiotic therapy obligatory)
4. Multiple renal cysts are a relative contraindication

For elective procedures:

- Patients advised to avoid diet (for 6 h) and fluids (for 4 h) prior to the procedure
- Ensuring the patient is ambulant will reduce intestinal gas
- Patients must also empty their bladder just before the procedure

- In the absence of urinary infection a single dose of an intravenous broad-spectrum antibiotic (e.g., cefuroxime 750 mg, or gentamicin 3–5 mg/kg) is adequate
- In patients with, or at risk of, uro-sepsis, antibiotics should be continued for at least 24 hours
- Patients are usually required to remain in prone position with a radiolucent pad/pillow under the abdomen to stabilize the kidney

The initial percutaneous renal puncture is performed under ultrasound guidance, fluoroscopy, or a combination of both. Although the majority of renal cannulation procedures are performed under local anesthesia, occasionally intravenous sedation or a general anesthetic will be required in the apprehensive or pediatric patient.

Renal puncture
- Initial skin incision
- Pelvicalyceal system is punctured using a long exploring 22 G needle (e.g., Kellet needle)
- It is important to avoid direct puncture of the renal pelvis due to risks of laceration, bleeding (without the tamponade effect of the parenchyma) and extravasation of urine
- Line of entry should be through the parenchyma, then into a calyx and then into the renal pelvis
- Urine aspiration will confirm correct placement
- Injection of contrast can provide additional verification
- Access is secured by the manipulation of a guidewire down the ureter
- The tract is dilated to allow placement of a suitable drainage catheter

Nephrostogram
- Can be performed immediately or deferred till the system has been adequately drained or in the presence of infection
- Between 50 and 100 mL of Urograffin 150 is used (but any HOCM or LOCM 150–200-strength media can be employed)
- Any residual contrast should be removed from an obstructed system to minimize risk of a chemical pyelitis
- Simple nephrostogram can be performed as an outpatient procedure, but overnight hospital stay is required if a percutaneous procedure has been performed

The effective radiation dose to the patient varies with the length of fluoroscopic exposure but usually ranges between 1 and 5 mSv.

Interpretation
Following injection of contrast, spot films are taken of the pelvicalyceal system and ureter down to the level of any obstruction. In some instances, dynamic fluouroscopic imaging can provide more pertinent information compared to a delayed review of hard copies. Images can be taken in the anterior or oblique position. Usually, nephrostomy imaging provides excellent quality images due to the lack of contrast dilution and the relatively small volume of the system under scrutiny.

* Intraluminal lesions are usually seen as filling defects. Filling defects with a smooth profile are more likely to represent stones, while irregular lesions are suggestive of malignancy
* Position and extent of strictured areas are clearly demonstrated. Smooth contours are indicative of extrinsic compression. Stricture formation secondary to intraluminal pathologies such as ureteric TCC are more liable to appear irregular in outline
* Obstruction can occur at any level within the upper urinary tract and is confirmed by proximal pooling of contrast with little or no distal flow

Whitaker test
This is a direct investigation of upper tract urodynamics if diuresis renography provides equivocal results. Following renal puncture, dilute contrast is infused in to the renal pelvis at a perfusion rate of 10 mL/min. Valid interpretation also requires simultaneous measurement of intravesical pressure. Interpretation is as follows:

* A pressure difference between upper and lower urinary tract of <15 cmH$_2$O excludes obstruction
* A pressure difference of more than 22 cmH$_2$O confirms obstruction
* A pressure difference of 15–22 cmH$_2$O lies in the equivocal range

Advantage
* Provides good anatomical information about the upper tract and the presence/nature of any obstruction

Drawbacks
- Requires the presence of a nephrostomy (invasive)
- Complications include—
  - Nephrostogram
    - ◊ Contrast allergy (less frequent than IV contrast)
    - ◊ Infection
    - ◊ Contrast extravasation
  - renal puncture
    - ◊ Failure to access kidney
    - ◊ Septicemia
    - ◊ Hemorrhage
    - ◊ Perforation of collecting system
    - ◊ Rarely, pneumothorax, hemothorax, bowel perforation

(h) RETROGRADE URETEROPYELOGRAPHY (RPG)

Overview
- RPG generally follows after an IVU, which has yielded insufficient results and persistent concerns require adequate demonstration of the pelvicalyceal system and the ureters
- The main advantage of RPG is that direct controlled injection of contrast media will allow satisfactory opacification of the upper tracts and therefore facilitates improved visualization of areas of concern, independent of renal impairment
- Main disadvantage is the need for cystoscopic insertion of ureteric catheters

Indications
- Demonstration of pelvicalyceal system after an inadequate IVU (especially if patient continues to have hematuria or abnormal urine cytology)
- Demonstrate site and extent of upper tract filling defect abnormality (e.g., stones, tumors, strictures) (Fig. 3.9)
- Assessment of ureteric anatomy (before ureteroscopic intervention or stent insertion; to exclude ureteric injury following upper tract endoscopic manipulation)
- As an alternative to IVU or CT if patient has renal impairment or allergy to intravenous contrast

Technique and radiation
This procedure is performed in conjunction with cystoscopy and will therefore require either sedation or general regional anes-

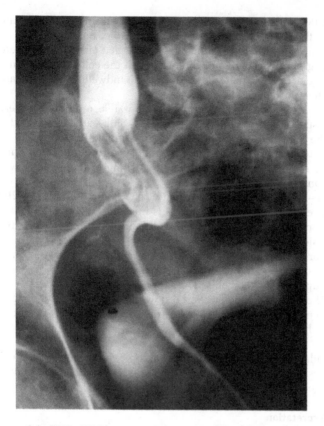

FIGURE 3.9. RPG—TCC lower ureter seen as a filling defect with caliber change (Courtesy of Dr A Bradley, Wythenshawe, Manchester)

thesia. Improved quality images are acquired if measures have been taken to minimise bowel related artifacts (e.g., avoid diet for 6–8 hours, aperients to minimize fecal loading, and patient to remain as ambulant as possible prior to surgery). The main contraindications are the presence of a UTI and pregnancy.

• All patients should receive a single prophylactic dose of a broad-spectrum intravenous antibiotic
• At cystoscopy, one or both ureters are catheterized by the urologist

- RPG can either be performed in the operating theater or later in the radiology department (better image quality)
- A 6 or 8 F ureteric catheter is positioned either in the ureter (e.g., below the area of interest) or in the collecting system
- The ureteric catheter is secured to an indwelling bladder catheter (for delayed imaging)
- If retrograde catheterization is not possible, or if lower ureteric visualization is required, a Braasch bulb catheter wedged in the ureteric orifice can be used for on-table RPG
- Before contrast injection, any air in the catheter lumen must be removed by aspiration or by flushing of the catheter with contrast
- 10–20 mL of Urograffin 150 (or HOCM or LOCM 150–200-strength water-soluble media) is injected slowly
- Contrast media may be diluted to avoid obscuring of small lesions
- Care must be taken not to cause contrast extravasation or bleeding due to overenthusiastic injecting
- Supine PA and/or oblique images are taken
- The ureteric catheter can be slowly withdrawn while imaging to perform a withdrawal ureterogram, or can be left in situ for a short period to drain

Similar to other dynamic fluoroscopic procedures, radiation exposure is related to length of fluoroscopy time, and usually ranges from 1 to 5 mSv.

Interpretation

The basic principles required to interpret nephrostomy images can be used in the interpretation of RPG images, except that contrast entry occurs in the opposite direction.

Advantages

- Good visualization of upper tract irrespective of renal function
- Decreased (but not zero) risk of contrast allergy

Drawbacks

- Invasive
- Often requires a general anesthesia
- Small lesions may be missed (false-negative rate up to 20%)
- Infection
- Contrast extravasation
- Ureteric trauma

(i) DOPPLER STUDIES

Overview
- Doppler technology is a useful adjunct to USS
- Technological advances have increased its utility in the real-time investigation
- The Doppler effect is a physical phenomenon which demonstrates a change in the frequency of a signal due to the relative movement of the signal source compared to the observer
- The Doppler signal is usually in the audible range
- Application of an ultrasound beam will allow the measurement of flow direction and velocity of any structure which moves (e.g., flow of RBC in a blood vessel)
- Simple continuous-wave Doppler can detect velocity but not depth of the signal source
- Pulsed Doppler, on the other hand, uses intermittent bursts of ultrasound and is capable of assessing depth as well as velocity and can adequately display the flow characteristics at a desired depth

The flow, direction, pulsatile rhythm, and resistivity of flow can be displayed either—

- Graphically (spectral trace)
- By color (color Doppler imaging)

Color Doppler imaging (CDI) is currently the technique of choice for the evaluation of blood flow and directional information in vessels and works by superimposing color over the conventional gray-scale image. Red demonstrates blood flow toward the transducer, while blue demonstrates flow away. CDI, however, is angle dependent and lacks sensitivity when imaging small, deep blood vessels or areas of slow blood flow.

Power Doppler imaging attempts to overcome the limitations of CDI, by displaying the amplitude (or strength) of the Doppler signal rather than simply the change in frequency. Power Doppler imaging works by detecting the density and movement of red blood cells and as such is independent of blood flow velocity and direction. It is 3–5 times more sensitive in the study of small, deep, slow-flowing blood vessels.

Dupplex scans combine real-time anatomic scanning with pulsed Doppler hemodynamic information and permits blood velocity estimation at different sites within a two-dimensional field.

In addition, recent reports using intravascular contrast agents which enhance the Doppler signal by the production of micro-bubbles have shown promising results in increasing sensitivity and reducing motion artifact. Advances in ultrasound and trans-ducer technology, though mostly experimental, are enabling higher-resolution imaging with 3D reconstruction and image manipulation of anatomical structures. Thus, in spite of signifi-cant advances in CT and MRI technology, Doppler-assisted ultra-sound is likely to remain an invaluable tool in the armamentarium of urological investigative methods for some time yet.

Indications
Some urological applications of Doppler studies are briefly described below:

- Kidney
  - Arterial or venous abnormalities (such as thrombosis, steno-sis, occlusion, aneurysm or fistula)
  - Calculation of the resistive index (RI) can help diagnose obstructive uropathy. An RI of >0.75 is indicative of obstruc-tion. The following calculation is used:

$$RI = \frac{\text{peak systolic velocity} - \text{lowest diastolic velocity}}{\text{peak systolic velocity}}$$

  - Assessment of vascularity of renal lesions
- Ureter: the absence of ureteric flow or jets on color Doppler is indicative of ureteric obstruction
- Bladder: in pediatric patients reflux of bladder urine into the ureter may suggest VUR
- Testis: Doppler sonography can visualize testicular blood flow and can assist in the diagnosis of torsion (absent flow) or acute inflammation (increased flow)
- Penis
  - Essential in the assessment of patients with ED, as it readily demonstrates penile vasculature, including the cavernosal arteries
  - Can help distinguish between high- and low-flow priapism

(j) CYSTOGRAM

Overview
- Cystography provides a more thorough examination of the bladder using direct contrast instillation

- Contrast media may be introduced in a retrograde fashion (via the urethra) or percutaneously (suprapubic bladder puncture)
- Cystography can be divided into three categories:
  1. Static (simple): this forms the bulk of the discussion in this chapter
  2. Dynamic: as part of urodynamic evaluation of the lower urinary tract (discussed in Chapter 5f—Videourodynamics)
  3. Micturating cystourethrography (MCUG): although this is discussed later in this book, the basics of technique will be described here

Indications

The general indications for direct contrast imaging of the bladder include—

- Bladder trauma
- Following open surgery on the bladder or prostate (e.g., augmentation cystoplasty, radical prostatectomy)
- Suspected vesical fistula
- Delineation of bladder diverticula
- Vesicoureteric reflux
- Urodynamic indications (e.g., stress incontinence, pelvic organ prolapse)

Technique and radiation

No specific patient preparation is required, although non-trauma patients must be asked to void before commencement of study. The main absolute contraindication to cystography is a UTI. Most children will receive antibiotic prophylaxis, although this is not routinely indicated in adults. In a patient with pelvic trauma, the integrity of the urethra must first be ascertained (using a retrograde urethrogram) prior to urethral catheterization. In such situations, cystography may still be carried out if safe suprapubic puncture of the bladder is possible.

- After a preliminary KUB, the bladder is catheterized
- Any water-soluble 150-strength contrast media can be used
- AP films must include bony landmarks (sacrum and symphysis pubis) to determine bladder neck descent
- In addition, 45° oblique and lateral views (with and without straining) should be taken, although this may not be possible in the pelvic trauma patient

Suspected bladder trauma

Ideally, a three-phase technique should be employed:

1. An initial 50 mL of contrast may demonstrate bladder rupture and no further contrast is required
2. If no abnormality is detected, a further 300 mL of contrast is instilled using a intravenous drip infusion giving set to adequately distend the bladder. Any significant breach of the bladder wall should become apparent
3. If cystogram remains normal, the bladder is emptied via the catheter and contrast extravasation from a small posterior tear may become obvious

Cystography following bladder surgery or for suspected vesical fistula

Typically up to 200 mL of contrast is instilled in the bladder of patients who have undergone open bladder/prostate surgery, 10–14 days post-operation. Evaluation of a fistula requires larger volumes of contrast (200–300 mL). Multiple-angle films can be obtained.

Micturating cystourethrography (MCUG)

MCUG is primarily performed in children with recurrent UTI suspected to have vesicoureteric reflux (VUR). MCUG also allows evaluation of the male (for urethral valves) and female (for urethral diverticula) urethra in pediatric patients.

- Residual urine is drained, recorded, and discarded
- Contrast can then be instilled via a giving set, under fluoroscopic control so any abnormal bladder activity or reflux can be identified
- Once the bladder is full, the catheter is removed and the patient encouraged to void under fluoroscopic visualization of the entire urinary tract
- Adults and older children can be placed in a vertical position to void into a container
- Smaller children and infants are encouraged to void lying down into an absorbent pad
- Suprapubic compression may be required for infants and neuropathic bladders to attain satisfactory elevation in the intravesical pressure for reflux to occur
- A final spot film of the bladder will help determine post-micturition residual volume

Modifications

A similar study can be performed using ^{99m}Tc-pertechnetate instilled into the bladder for the diagnosis of VUR in children. Gamma camera detection of radioactivity is carried out throughout the study. The main advantage is the significantly reduced radiation dose to the patient, but this is at the expense of anatomical detail.

Recent reports have demonstrated a superior rate of bladder trauma detection using CT cystogram. Following instillation of 300–350 mL of contrast, CT scanning can be performed with a full and then empty bladder. This is an attractive option if the trauma patient is already on the CT scan table for suspected other abdominal trauma, and does not need to be transferred to another room.

Interpretation

Interpretation of the MCUG is discussed in chapter 11 on the investigation of the pediatric patient with hydronephrosis. The discussion here will be confined to the patient with bladder injury.

Pelvic fractures are complicated by bladder rupture in 5–10% of cases and static cystography (or CT cystography) diagnoses the rupture in virtually all cases, providing adequate distension of the bladder with contrast has occurred. A blood clot or omental flap may temporarily plug a small tear and cause this to be overlooked.

Classification of injuries

1. *Pelvic hematoma*: occasionally even in the absence of any direct bladder trauma, the bladder outline might be distorted due to the presence of a pelvic hematoma. The bladder may either appear pushed to one side, or appear elongated, ovoid in shape, and pushed up out of the pelvis ("teardrop" bladder) due to bilateral compression from the hematoma. CT cystography will readily demonstrate the hematoma.

2. *Bladder contusion and interstitial rupture (non-full-thickness tear)*: these account for about a third of all traumatic bladder injuries and are generally diagnoses of exclusion. No contrast extravasation is noted, but part of the bladder outline may appear irregular and distorted.

3. *Extraperitoneal rupture*: rupture usually occurs on the antero-lateral bladder wall and is almost exclusively seen in pelvic fractures, as the bladder base is sheared by distortion of

the pelvic ring. Perivesical contrast leakage results in streaky, flame-shaped extravasation, which may extend into the anterior wall, inguinal region, and upper thigh area. Breach of the urogential diaphragm could result in contrast within the perineum and scrotum. It is important to note the presence of bony spikes which may have penetrated the bladder wall.

4. *Intraperitoneal rupture*: accounts for about 10–20% of bladder rupture and sudden increased intravesical pressure tends to cause rupture at the weakest and most mobile part of the bladder, the dome. A diffuse distribution of contrast within the peritoneum can be seen with outlining of bowel loops. Intraperitoneal bladder rupture occurs more frequently in children due to the intraperitoneal position of the pediatric bladder. Surgical exploration and repair are mandatory.

5. *Intra- and extraperitoneal rupture*: both types of injuries may coexist in around 10% of cases. Cystography findings are a combination of the two pathologies.

In non-trauma patients (e.g., following open bladder or pelvic surgery), contrast noted outside the lumen of the lower urinary tract is indicative of local anastamotic leakage. Vesico-vaginal and vesico-enteric fistulae can be readily diagnosed with static cystography, but MRI may be used in equivocal cases.

Advantage
- Very useful for assessment of bladder anatomy and function (especially in children)

Drawbacks
- Involves radiation
- Invasive
- Risk of infection
- Contrast extravasation may result in local inflammation

(k) URETHROGRAPHY

Overview
- The most common radiological investigation for the evaluation of the male and female urethra
- Frequency of urethrography is decreasing due to improved endoscopic techniques
- Provides superior anatomical information
- Performed via the antegrade (micturating cystourethrography—MCUG) or the retrograde (ascending) approach

- Antegrade approach is better for visualization of the posterior urethra
- Retrograde approach is the procedure of choice for anterior urethral studies
- Some patients can be imaged using both techniques
- Dynamic technique (i.e., imaging during contrast movement through the urethra) provides the most clinically pertinent data

Indications

- Strictures (post-inflammatory or post-traumatic) (Fig. 3.10b,c)
- Urethral trauma (secondary to penile, pelvic, or iatrogenic trauma)
- Urethral diverticulum (mainly in females)
- Fistulae or false passages (Fig. 3.10a)
- Peri-urethral or prostatic abscess
- Congenital abnormalities
- Urethral tumors (primarily to assess luminal patency and not for staging)

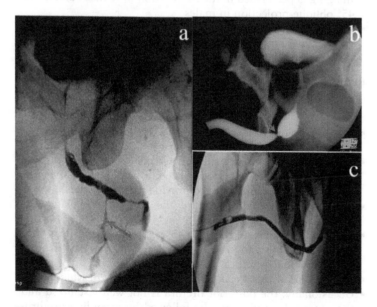

FIGURE 3.10. Urethrography—(**a**) severe distal penile urethral stricture with formation of urethro-cutaneous fistula formation (arrow), (**b**) bulbar urethral stricture (**c**) full-length stricture (Courtesy of Mr S Payne, Manchester Royal Infirmary)

Technique and radiation

The main contraindication is the presence of a concurrent UTI. In addition, due to edema and risk of subsequent scarring following instrumentation, contrast studies are best deferred for at least 6 weeks post-surgery.

- The patient is asked to void just before the study
- The use of prophylactic antibiotics is discretionary
- Any pre-warmed, 200–300-strength HOCM or LOCM may be used, 30 mL is usually sufficient for retrograde studies, while MCUG will typically use 200–300 mL

MCUG study of the urethra is rarely indicated in adults, but if required the following technique is used:

- 200 mL of contrast is instilled into the bladder
- The patient is asked to void under screening
- Imaging is performed in the AP position in females and in the 45° oblique projection in males
- Urethral distension can be enhanced by asking the patient to void against resistance (e.g., penile clamp)

Retrograde studies are virtually confined to males and usually provide excellent demonstration of the entire urethra.

- A 2–16 F Foley catheter is inserted 2 cm into the urethra to sit in the fossa navicularis
- The catheter balloon is distended with 2 mL of water to provide a seal. If the balloon is not utilized, a penile clamp over the penile tip can be employed to provide external occlusion
- Contrast is injected slowly till the base of the bladder is outlined
- Images are usually taken in the 45° right oblique position with the patient's hip and knee slightly flexed, as this best demonstrates the male urethra
- AP and lateral views can be helpful, especially in women
- Occasionally, the posterior urethra is not well visualized and the antegrade study must be followed by a voiding urethrogram. Some urethral fistulas and diverticulum, periurethral abscesses, and reflux into prostatic duct are best demonstrated during voiding of contrast

Interpretation

Congenital urethral valves: posterior valves are the most common congenital urethral anomaly in males and are usually diagnosed in early childhood. These are best demonstrated on MCUG and classically appear as well-defined linear filling defects obstructing contrast flow, with proximal dilatation of the prostatic urethra.

Urethral diverticulum: occurs more commonly in females (acquired) but can be seen in males (congenital). In females, the most common location is the mid-urethra, in a postero-lateral position and is seen as a contrast-filled smooth, rounded sac attached to the urethra by a short neck. Congenital diverticula in males occur along the ventral aspect of the mid-penile urethra.

Urethral trauma: trauma to the urethra is effectively restricted to males. Debate exists as to the timing of contrast study. Traditionally, any patient with a suspected urethral injury would undergo urethrography at time of initial presentation in order to classify the site and extent of damage. Advocates of the delayed technique (3–6 months later) argue that the acute-phase study is unlikely to affect initial patient management, and moreover, a subsequent urethrogram will be required in order to assess the anatomical and stricture status of the urethra prior to considering surgical repair.

Nevertheless, posterior urethral injuries can be classified according to their urethrographic appearances and are summarized below (see Table 3.7).

Trauma to the anterior urethra is usually secondary to urethral instrumentation or blunt perineal trauma. Urethrogram often demonstrates contrast extravasation into the corpora spongiosum. Complete ruptures are indicated by an abrupt end to the contrast in the urethra.

Strictures: inflammatory strictures usually occur at the proximal bulbar urethra; may be multiple with varying lengths; and may demonstrate contrast within the periurethral glands. If severe, urethroperineal fistulae may be seen. Traumatic (including iatrogenic) strictures are seen around the bulbomembranous area; are usually solitary; and often short (<2 cm). Complete demonstration of a tight stricture may be a combined retrograde and antegrade (suprapubic) urethrogram.

TABLE 3.7. Posterior urethral injuries classified according to their urethrographic appearances

Type	Description	Contrast Pattern
I (mild)	Contusion or partial tear of the urethra The urethra may be stretched and narrowed due to bladder elevation by pelvic hematoma	No extravasation
II (most common)	Rupture of the urethra just above the urogenital diaphragm (prostatic apex); the bulbar urethra is intact	Contrast extravasation seen in the retropubic space but *not* into the perineum; two-thirds are complete tears and no contrast is seen in the bladder; contrast within the bladder following retrograde study is indicative of a partial rupture
III (severe)	Rupture of the membranous urethra, below the urogenital diaphragm, at the bulbomembranous junction	Contrast extravasation is seen in the perineum and *not* the retropubic space, virtually all type III ruptures are complete, so no bladder filling will be seen

As a general rule complete tears—

- Occur twice as often as partial tears
- Stricture more often
- Require open surgical repair

Partial ruptures, on the other hand, are usually treated conservatively with catheterization

Others: urethral tumors can be seen as smooth or irregular filling defects, with or without associated stricture formation. Periurethral and periprostatic abscesses are best demonstrated on voiding urethrography.

Advantage
• Accurate visualization of urethral anatomy

Drawbacks
• Introduction of infection
• Catheter-related urethral trauma
• Use of excessive force can result in contrast extravasation
• Contrast allergic reactions (but rare)

(I) CAVERNOSOGRAPHY

Overview
• Cavernosography (and cavernosometry) can be used to evaluate venous problems in men with ED
• The increased use of penile duplex Doppler techniques have significantly restricted their use
• These methods are often reserved for patients who have previously undergone a "normal" set of non-invasive ultrasonographic investigations

In the normal individual, appropriate stimulation results in smooth muscle relaxation of the arteriolar inflow into the corpora cavernosa. Simultaneous venous outflow occlusion is essential to the maintenance of a full erection, and abnormal venous leakage (estimated to be the cause of ED in at least 25% of patients) can be demonstrated by dynamic infusion cavernosometry and cavernosography.

Indications
Although non-invasive methods have now become the mainstay of erectile function assessment, the traditional indications for direct infusion and contrast cavernosal studies include—

• Assessment of vasculogenic ED if considering surgery
• Investigation of priapism (high flow)
• Assessment of penile fractures/injury to assess cavernosal damage
• Assessment of Peyronie's disease (rarely used)

Technique and interpretation

This study is usually performed as an outpatient procedure and no specific patient preparation is required. The only absolute contraindication is a previous history of contrast allergy.

Cavernosometry

- Two 19–22 G butterfly needles are inserted into the corpora. Care must be taken to avoid perforation of the urethra
- An erection is induced by an intracorporeal injection of 10–20 µg of prostaglandin E_1
- One of the needles is used to record intracavernosal pressures. A record is made of any increase in pressure up to the maximum pressure and the time taken to achieve it. A normal response is indicated by the intracavernosal pressure approaching mean arterial blood pressure within 5–10 minutes. Failure to do so may either be due to impaired inflow or increased outflow
- If after 10 minutes, there is no erection or the pressure is <80 mmHg, an infusion of saline (100–200 mL/min) is commenced via the other needle
- Erection should be achieved within 3 minutes; if not, the procedure should be concluded due to risks of local edema and systemic fluid overload
- A record is kept of the rate of infusion required to attain a full erection (normally less than 120 mL/min)
- Once a full erection is reached, the infusion is stopped and a note made of the rate of pressure drop. In normal patients this should be less than 1.5 mmHg and a rapid decline is indicative of a venous leak. The saline infusion can also be slowly recommenced to produce a flow adequate to maintain a full erection. Maintenance flow rates of >15 mL/s are suggestive of a venous leak. If a venous leak is suggested, cavernosography is performed

For cavernosography

- A contrast media (60–100 mL of Omnipaque or urograffin) is infused slowly to obtain a pressure in the penis of 90 mmHg, which is physiologic pressure
- If the penis is not erect, contrast leakage into the veins is inevitable and therefore a full erection is mandatory
- Dynamic fluoroscopy should include AP and right and left oblique views. Under normal circumstances, no contrast should be visualized outside the two, near-straight corpora cavernosa (see Fig 3.11a,b). Any areas of contrast leakage or significant curvature are abnormal

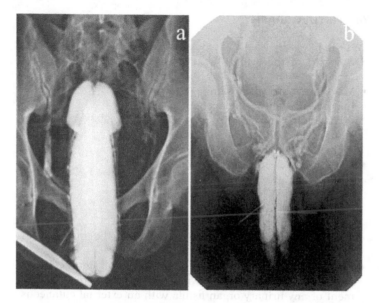

FIGURE 3.11. Cavernosogram—(a) normal, (b) gross bilateral venous leakage with no evidence of tumescence (Courtesy of Mr S Payne, Manchester Royal Infirmary)

- On completion of the study, the needles are removed to allow resolution of the erection
- The patient is also advised to squeeze the penis for 5 min to ensure complete emptying. Rarely, a priapism may occur, requiring incremental doses of ephedrine to accomplish detumescence

Pathological venous leakage is demonstrated by contrast in the superficial or deep dorsal veins, cavernosal veins and crural veins (in increasing degrees of clinical significance).

Advantage
- More sensitive and accurate in demonstrating venous leakage (compared to Doppler techniques)

Drawbacks
- Invasive
- Can be painful
- Risk of infection
- Theoretical risk of contrast related fibrosis within the corpora
- Risk of priapism

(m) FISTULOGRAPHY

Overview
- Any part of the urinary tract can be involved in a fistulous process
- May break through to skin
- Imaging modality will depend on—
  - The anatomical site
  - Function of the urinary organ involved
  - The precise information required
- Fistulous tracks may result from
  - Infections
  - Inflammation
  - Malignancy
  - Surgical trauma
- Cross-sectional imaging (MRI and CT) is the mainstay of imaging
- Fistulography (by inserting a blunt needle or small catheter into the mouth of the fistula) may play a role in the management of any urinary organ fistula with an external cutaneous connection (e.g., renocutaneous, ureterocutaneous, enterocutaneous, vesicocutaneous, or urethrocutaneous fistulae)

Indications
- Indicated in any existing or suspected fistula with a cutaneous opening
- The purpose is to demonstrate opacification of pathological tracks or extravasation of contrast medium from hollow organs

Technique
Fistulography must be avoided in the presence of significant sepsis and should be delayed in high-output fistulas till the traffic decreases. No specific patient preparation is required in most cases.

- Choice of catheter is determined by the bore of the track, and catheters ranging from thin sialography cannulae to large Foley catheters may be used
- Ideally, either the catheter itself or catheter balloon should occlude fistula opening, avoid leakage and allow sufficient filling pressure
- A water-soluble contrast medium is injected under fluoroscopic control, although barium may be used if bowel opacification is desired

- Spot filming should include a minimum of two radiographs at right angles
- When examining complex tracks, a catheter with sideholes is advantageous

Fistulography can help—

- Determine the site of origin of fistula
- Demonstrate a communication into abscess
- Confirm the presence or absence of distal obstruction

A direct fistulogram may often be more appropriate in cases of renocutaneous fistulas, since contrast CT images are often compromised by a potentially non-functioning kidney. More recently, fistulography has been combined with CT to allow improved anatomical demonstration of the underlying pathology in complex disease. In addition, saline fistulography followed by MR imaging has been shown to give even better soft tissue resolution than CT due to the multiplanar capabilities of MRI. Recent studies using hydrogen peroxide ultrasound fistulography in bowel-related fistula have shown fistula tract visualization as good as that achieved with the direct contrast technique. In this method, 20–90 mL of the peroxide solution (30% hydrogen peroxide and 70% povidone/iodine) is slowly injected into the fistula and the production of gas bubbles aids USS localization.

Chapter 4
Nuclear Medicine Investigations

Introduction

Nuclear medicine techniques are integral to modern urological practice and can be used to investigate almost any organ in the body. Urological usage is primarily confined to—

- Assessment of renal imaging, function, and drainage
- Management of metastatic prostate cancer

Isotopes of an element share the same atomic number (and therefore the same biochemical characteristics) but differ in their mass number (as well as their energy states). An example is the isotopes of iodine (^{123}I, ^{131}I, ^{125}I). When an isotope has radioactive properties, it is called a radioisotope or radionuclide. Radionuclides undergo spontaneous disintegration, while emitting high—penetrating, electromagnetic gamma rays (measured in electron volts [eV]). Radionuclides are used to label a compound, with a specific interaction with the target organ (e.g., kidney, bone) and the resulting ionizing radiation is detected and quantified by a gamma camera. A nuclear medicine image, therefore, is a map of where the tracer has accumulated, and is dependent on blood flow to the target organ as well as tracer metabolism by the organ (an indicator of function).

The characteristics of the three main radionuclides used in urological practice are summarized in Table 4.1.

The half-life of a radiopharmaceutical (radionuclide + labeled compound) is determined by its natural rate of nuclide decay and metabolism/handling by the body. Decay is measured in Becquerals (Bq) and 1 Bq equals 1 disintegration per second. Typically, diagnostic procedures result in a dose delivery of 10^6 Bq (1 MBq) and therapeutic interventions in 10^9 Bq (1 GBq). The ideal radiopharmaceutical should have the following characteristics:

TABLE 4.1. Radionuclides

Radionuclide	Isotopes	Half-Life	Energy of Gamma Rays (keV)	Labeled Compounds
Technetium-99m	^{99m}Tc	6.02 h	140	DTPA DMSA MAG3
Iodine	^{123}I, ^{131}I, ^{125}I	13.2 h (^{123}I)	159	Hippuran
Chromium	^{51}Cr	27.7 days	320	EDTA

1. Easily and cheaply generated
2. Radiochemically pure
3. Non-toxic
4. Should emit only gamma rays (100–200 keV energy)
5. Half-life long enough to complete investigation
6. Half-life short enough to minimize patient radiation risk

Table 4.2 describes the characteristics of the commonly used radiopharmaceutical.

Therefore, nuclear medicine techniques in renography can evaluate—

• Renal blood flow
• Renal cortical imaging
• Renal glomerular filtration
• Renal handling
• Renal excretion

The agent of choice will primarily depend on the precise function being evaluated.

Positron emission tomography (PET) is an emerging radio-nuclide technique which has recently enjoyed a migration from the research setting into clinical practice. The most commonly used radionuclide in PET scanning is fluorine-18 which binds to a D-glucose analog. The basic principles of PET and possible application in urology are discussed in Chapter 4e.

In general, radiopharmaceuticals—

• Are safe in the short term
• Rarely cause allergic reactions

TABLE 4.2. Commonly used radiopharmaceuticals in urology practice

Radionuclide	Radiopharmaceutical	Half-life	Injected adults dose (MBq)	Effective dose (mSv)	Characteristics	Applications
Technitium-99m	Dimercaptosuccinic acid (^{99m}Tm-DMSA)	6.02 h	1/kg body weight (max dose 80)	1	All activity in plasma with strong binding to plasma proteins; not filtered by glomerulus; slow extraction of DMSA from blood into proximal tubule cells; bound to cytoplasmic proteins and mitochondria within cells; tracer accumulation within both proximal and distal tubules	Renal imaging

Most accurate measurement of split renal function |
| | Diethylenetriamine pentaacetic acid (^{99m}Tm-DTPA) | 6.02 h | 10–300

10 for GFR estimation 50–75 for renography | 1 | Slowly cleared by glomerular filtration; cheap and easy to produce; poor target-to-background ratio in poor renal function | GFR estimation

Renography |

Compound	Half-life	Dose		Comments	Use
Mercaptoacetyltriglycine (^{99m}Tm-MAG3)	6.02 h	50–100 50–100 for renography	3	Cleared by tubular secretion and glomerular filtration	Renography Estimation of ERPF
Methylene diphosphonate (^{99m}Tm-medronate)	6.02 h	800	8	High uptake of immature bone results in increased tracer uptake in areas of rapid bone turnover	Bone imaging
Iodine Orthoiodohippurate (^{123}I-Hippuran)	13.2 h	20–75 20 for renography 2 for ERPF	0.3	Hippuran has best clearance of all tracers; fast renal handling; eliminated mainly by tubular secretion and glomerular filtration; expensive	^{123}I—ideal for renography ^{125}I and ^{131}I best for ERPF
Chromium Ethylenediamine tetraacetic acid (^{51}Cr-EDTA)	27.7 days	3	0.007	Stable compound which is cleared by glomerular filtration; not widely available	GFR estimation

- Have long-term risks common to all forms of radiation, including development of malignancies and genetic injury which may be inheritable. A safe level of radiation does not exist and all exposure must be kept as low as reasonably achievable (**ALARA** principle)
- Ought to be avoided in pregnant and lactating women unless in exceptional circumstances. Since most radiopharmaceuticals are excreted in breast milk, lactating mothers are advised to stop nursing for 2–3 days
- Are excreted primarily in urine and patients must be advised to urinate frequently post-examination to minimize radiation risk
- When given to pediatric patients must be dose adjusted for body weight of patient

Clinical applications

A discussion of all radionuclide clinical applications and their techniques is beyond the scope and purpose of this book and the authors will limit the discussion to the following categories:

(a) MAG3 renography
(b) DMSA scan
(c) Obtaining a GFR
(d) Bone scan
(e) PET scan
(f) Detection of prostate cancer metastases

(a) MAG3 RENOGRAPHY

Overview

^{99m}Tc-MAG3 has become the agent of choice for dynamic radionuclide imaging of the renal tract in most centers. It was first developed as an alternative to hippuran, but has a plasma clearance 50–65% slower than that of hippuran. Nevertheless, it gives images comparable to ^{123}I-hippuran. Following intravenous injection, it remains loosely bound to serum proteins, and only a small proportion undergoes glomerular filtration. Clearance is predominantly by tubular secretion. The 30-minute excretion of ^{99m}Tc-MAG3 is approximately 70%, and by 3 hours 90% of the tracer is cleared by the kidneys. Renography can be combined with administration of a diuretic (usually frusemide) to produce a high urine flow diuresis renogram. The ^{99m}Tc-MAG3 is an adequate tool for the assessment of urinary uptake, transit, excretion, and split renal function. In addition, simple conversion methods will allow reproducible estimations of ERPF from the ^{99m}Tc-MAG3 activity curve.

Indications
- Assessment of whole or relative kidney function
  - Before and after surgical intervention (e.g., pyeloplasty, partial/total nephrectomy)
  - Investigation of acute or chronic renal failure
  - Assessment of the transplanted kidney
  - Assessment of renal function following trauma
- Assessment of kidney drainage in obstructive uropathy (e.g., uretero-pelvic junction obstruction, renal stones)
- Assessment of congenital renal abnormalities (e.g., dupplex, horseshoe, absent, ectopic, or cystic kidneys)
- Identification of vesico-ureteric reflux

Technique and radiation
The Consensus Committee of the Society of Radionuclides in Nephrourology (1994) have published guidelines aimed at standardizing the renography protocol in order to enhance uniformity and reproducibility. These are summarized below.

Patient preparation
- Adequate hydration (500 mL of oral fluid 15–30 min before examination) is vital to ensure good diuresis (urine flow of 1–3 mL/min). Avoid study if patient appears clinically dehydrated
- The patient may be placed supine or erect, reclining against the camera
- Assess need for catheterization. If not, patient must void before study
- Position patient in either supine or sitting up position. The posture of the patient may have an effect on the renography curve (discussed later)
- A typical adult dose of 50–120 MBq is carefully injected intravenously to avoid local extravasation
- An image is taken every 10–20 seconds for up to 40 minutes following administration of radiopharmaceutical
- Analog images are taken every 5 minutes and the hard copy must include several serial analog images as well as the renogram curve
- The first 12 and last 12 frames may be summed to exhibit the kidneys more clearly
- If the kidney fails to empty by 20 minutes, frusemide may be administered (F+20). Data is collected for 30–45 minutes (or 20 min following diuretic injection)

- The patient is asked to void at the end of the procedure (minimizes radiation to the bladder as well as allowing assessment of urine production rate)
- The renogram curve demonstrates change in kidney activity over time

The radiation activity detected by the gamma camera is first stored as a computer image. Regions of interest (ROI) are mapped out for the kidneys and bladder, in addition to a background region to enable precise measurement of activity count for each time frame. The background region is usually chosen just lateral to the kidneys, but care must be taken to avoid the liver, due to its high tracer uptake. Additional ROIs (different moieties of a dupplex kidney) may also be delineated. The renogram curve can be obtained following subtraction of the background count from the kidney and bladder ROI count and is displayed as a percentage of the injected dose (y-axis) against time (x-axis). The relative function of each kidney is calculated by comparing the percentage dose at 2 and 3 minutes' uptake.

Following the procedure, the patient is informed about the possibility of a prolonged diuresis. Frequent voids will help reduce bladder irradiation.

Diuresis
If diuresis renography is indicated, an intravenous bolus of frusemide (dose 1 mg/kg in infants, 0.5 mg/kg in children aged 1–16 years, and 40 mg in adults) is commonly used. Ensure there are no contraindications to diuretic therapy. Frusemide will produce a maximal diuretic response within 5–10 minutes and rationale is to increase the sensitivity of the dynamic renal study by increasing urine flow rates to stress the system, such that minor degrees of obstruction are unmarked. The timing of diuretic administration is a matter of local policy but the various techniques have distinct advantages. The traditional technique (F+20) involves frusemide administration 20 minutes after injection of the radiopharmaceutical. The study must continue for at least 20 minutes following frusemide injection. This enables study of initial unmodified renal handling, followed by the response to increased urine flow rate.

The F-15 technique (frusemide given 15 min before radiopharmaceutical) ensures maximal diuresis at commencement of data acquisition, thereby revealing minor levels of obstruction. Administration of the tracer simultaneously with frusemide (F+0 technique) has been practised in pediatric units and has the advantage of significantly reducing examination times. The F+0 technique is not recommended in patients with significant renal failure (GFR < 15 mL/min per kidney) and renal units with significant hydronephrosis.

The timing of diuretic does not significantly alter split renal function result, but centers should standardize practice to enable meaningful comparisons (e.g., before and after surgical intervention). The F-15 technique will separate the majority of equivocal curves on F+20 renography in to either unobstructed or obstructed, and therefore is preferred in patients with equivocal results or with gross hydronephrosis.

Factors influencing MAG3 renography

1. Renal function: a GFR of <15 mL/min per single kidney will result in urine flow rates of <10 mL/min, with poor subsequent tracer washout. This may result in an "obstructed" (false-positive) curve. Frusemide is usually insufficient to increase diuresis significantly and perfusion pressure-flow studies (Whitaker test) ought to be considered. Renal disease affecting the parenchyma (e.g., acute tubular necrosis) may diminish the response to diuretics.

2. Hydration: minor levels of obstruction may be masked in dehydrated individuals. In addition, diuretic administration may be perilous if the patient is already dehydrated. Oral hydration (500 mL of water 30 min before study) will usually suffice although on occasions intravenous fluids may be required.

3. Collecting system capacity: in the massively dilated system, urine flow may be inadequate to prevent tracer accumulation in the renal pelvis. In such cases, a false-positive "obstructed" curve may be the end result. The F-15 technique will help minimize the effects of a capacious system.

4. Collecting system compliance: increased diuresis, within a normo-compliant system, should result in distension of the renal pelvis with no significant increase in pressure. However, poor compliance may cause rapid elevations within a non-dilated system, such that any obstruction is overcome and there is reasonable tracer flow distal to the obstruction (false negative). Conversely, a hyper-compliant upper tract will result in renal pelvic tracer accumulation, in spite of the absence of obstruction, resulting in a false-positive curve.

5. Bladder effects: a full bladder may inhibit drainage from the ureters and cause artifacts. The patient must be asked to void prior to commencement and again before completion of data acquisition. Alternatively, in patients with chronic retention or a neurogenic bladder, catheterization should abolish any effects of a full bladder.

6. Ureteric dilatation or obstruction: in cases of gross ureteric dilatation, an ROI drawn around the kidney and renal pelvis may miss the distal obstruction, resulting in a false-negative study. Care must be taken to study the analog images and ROI must include the ureter proximal to the obstruction. Furthermore, multiple simultaneous levels of obstruction will not be apparent by MAG3 renography.

The maximal recommended activity per test is 100 MBq for MAG3 renography, which corresponds to an effective radiation dose of 1 mSv (equivalent to 6 months of background radiation).

Interpretation

Normal renogram curve
The shape of the renogram curve (following subtraction of background activity) is dependent on—

1. MAG3 uptake from blood into kidney
2. MAG3 elimination from kidney into bladder

Classically, the normal MAG3 renogram curve has three phases (see figure 4.1):

- The first phase: steep upward rise following intravenous contrast injection; this is indicative of the speed of tracer injection and its delivery to the kidneys (i.e., renal vascular supply)
- The second phase: a more gradual slope which represents renal handling of MAG3 (renal uptake by tubular secretion and glomerular filtration) and peaks between 2 and 5 minutes. Time taken for the curve to peak following tracer injection is referred to as Tmax. This may be delayed in patients with renovascular insufficiency, renal failure, and obstruction
- The third phase: commences after the peak. Associated with the emergence of tracer in the bladder. Represents elimination (but also delivery) of tracer from the kidney. After 3 minutes

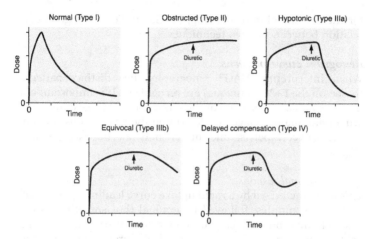

FIGURE 4.1. MAG3—Renography curve patterns in F + 20 diuresis renography (with permission from *Comprehensive Urology*, Weiss, Mosby, 2001, **141**)

both elimination and uptake are in competition, but the former subsequently dominates. It is this elimination curve that is dependent on the upper tract urodynamics. The elimination curve may have a smooth or stepwise (variant of normal) pattern and when normal, excludes the presence of obstruction. A delayed upward deflection may indicate intermittent obstruction or vesico-ureteric reflux

Split renal function
This is expressed as the ratio of the area under the renogram curves of the two kidneys obtained during the period 40 seconds to 2 minutes 40 seconds after tracer injection. The shortest transit time for filtrate in the Bowman's capsule to the renal pelvis is 2.5 minutes, and therefore it can be safely assumed that the MAG3 will not be found in the collecting system within 2.5 minutes of injection. The initial 40 seconds are excluded to prevent artifactual errors. The relative function in a pair of normally working kidneys may vary between 40% and 60%. Similarly, relative functions in different moieties of a dupplex kidney can also be calculated.

Scarring
Since 80% of MAG3 is metabolized by tubular secretion, the analog images can be analyzed for the presence of parenchymal scarring. Although DMSA renography remains the gold standard

for the investigation of scarring, MAG3 studies show good correlation between the two techniques.

Renogram curve patterns

When interpreting MAG3 renography, five distinct patterns (based on the F+20 technique) are recognized. It is important not merely to assess the shape of the curve, but also to examine the sequential analog images to determine the level of obstruction, as the calyces, pelvis, and ureter may all be easily visible (Fig. 4.1).

Type I—normal response

This is characterized by a rapid uptake curve leading up to a peak within 2–5 minutes, followed by gradual (but sometimes stepwise) elimination of tracer. Administration of frusemide results in no appreciable difference in speed of elimination. A normal curve virtually excludes obstruction, although it may be argued that increasing urine flow rate (i.e., using the F-15 technique) may expose lesser degrees of impedance.

Type II—obstructive response (high-pressure system)

In the absence of any other factors affecting drainage (e.g., dehydration, renal impairment, etc.), an obstructive pattern is denoted by a rising curve. In addition, the lack of an exponential tracer elimination curve is also suggestive of a degree of obstruction. Typically, there is little or no response to frusemide. On the analog images, the affected kidney will often display good parenchymal uptake and accumulation of tracer above the level of obstruction (e.g., in the renal pelvis in patients with UPJO). The diagnosis of obstruction cannot be satisfactorily made (even in the presence of a rising curve) if the affected kidney has a GFR of <15 mL/min, since the rate of urine production may be insufficient to produce tracer washout (usually 1–3 mL/min urine production is required).

Type IIIa—dilated but not obstructed (low pressure/
  hypotonic system)

There is an initial accumulation of tracer in the kidney, resulting in a rising curve similar to an obstructive response, but there is prompt elimination following frusemide injection. The analog images usually demonstrate tracer accrual in a dilated system secondary to stasis rather than obstruction. The increased urine flow produced by the diuretic is adequate to effect free drainage.

Type IIIb—equivocal response
Following an initial "obstructed" rising curve, a frusemide injection produces a somewhat languid response. The curve demonstrates some tendency to washout, albeit incompletely. Examination of the analog images may help clarify whether this represents partial obstruction or inadequate tracer elimination (e.g., due to a dilated renal pelvis). In this situation, an F-15 study will help categorize the majority of equivocal curves into either obstructed or non-obstructed.

Type IV—delayed compensation (Homsy's sign)
Described by Yves Homsy in 1988, the characteristic shape is a "double peak" response to diuretic. This pattern is seen in patients with subclinical intermittent obstruction. A repeat F-15 diuresis renography will often reveal an obstructed pattern. The first "peak" is due to an initial rising curve, which then exhibits a good response to frusemide. However, as the diuretic effect increases, the threshold is reached and tracer accumulation causes the curve to either flatten or rise.

Modifications of the MAG3 renography

Deconvolution analysis
This is a mathematical manipulation of the renogram to produce a theoretical curve that would be derived if the tracer had been injected in the renal artery (rather than a peripheral vein). This allows calculation of a range of transit times through the renal tubules, including mean parenchymal transit time as well as whole kidney transit time. Transit times are increased in obstruction and renal failure. Attention to technical detail is paramount, and as yet deconvolution techniques have not gained widespread acceptance.

Captopril-enhanced renography
This modification is indicated for the investigation of renal artery stenosis. Patients should be instructed to stop any angiotensin-converting enzyme (ACE) inhibitor or diuretics for at least 3 days prior to examination. Ensure patient is well hydrated. A baseline study is performed first. Following this, a further study is repeated (on the same day or consecutive days) with 25 mg of Captopril (ACE inhibitor) given orally 1 hour before tracer injection. Renin converts angiotensinogen to angiotensin I, which in turn is converted (by an ACE) into angiotensin II. Angiotensin II effects efferent arteriole vasoconstriction and thereby maintains GFR.

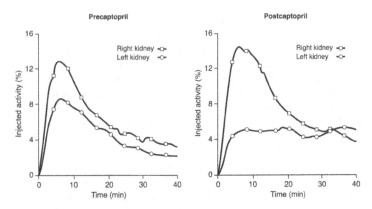

FIGURE 4.2. Captopril renography demonstrating a left renal artery sterosis (with permission from *Comprehensive Urology*, Weiss, Mosby, 2001, **145**)

Patients with reno-vascular (e.g., renal artery) stenosis have higher levels of angiotensin II. The captopril-enhanced renogram therefore will display reduced function (reduced gradient in the uptake part of the curve) and delayed transit, with a delay in T_{max} (time taken for renogram curve to peak) (see fig 4.2). The overall sensitivity of this technique is 80–90% for the detection of reno-vascular hypertension, and patients with positive results can often be successfully treated.

Renal transplant evaluation

MAG3 renography is non-nephrotoxic and a vital tool in the assessment of renal transplant patients. Clinical applications include—

- Pre-transplant evaluation of renal function and drainage in the potential living related donor
- In the immediate post-transplant period, serial MAG3 studies can help distinguish between a variety of potential pathologies:
  - Within the first 4 weeks, renography demonstrating no tracer uptake is usually indicative of a renal perfusion disorder (renal artery stenosis or renal vein thrombosis) or acute rejection
  - Diminished uptake of tracer with delayed and sluggish drainage is typical of acute tubular nephrosis or urinary tract obstruction (renal perfusion is usually maintained)

- With serial renography, a deterioration of function over time is indicative of rejection
- Renal outflow obstruction (e.g., at the ureterovesical junction) can be diagnosed easily
- Locations of urinary leakage and urinoma formation are readily identified

Indirect micturating cystography

Practice of this technique, which negates the use of a catheter, has many advantages in the pediatric population:

- Will primarily demonstrate reflux
- Enables estimation of split renal function
- Demonstrates cortical scarring
- Measures drainage
- Allows valuable assessment of bladder function

The well-hydrated patient is injected with an MAG3 tracer. If renography is required, data collection can commence immediately. The patient is then asked to void 30–60 minutes following tracer injection as data acquisition continues. An upward deflection in one or both of the kidney curves is suggestive of VUR. The main disadvantages are the prerequisite for children to be potty trained and the lack of anatomical detail. Unfortunately, this technique is associated with a high false-negative rate, especially for milder grades of reflux.

Advantages of MAG3 renography
- Provides sensitive indices of tubular function and urinary excretion
- Virtually no contraindications
- Non-nephrotoxic
- No significant risk of allergic reactions
- Serial examinations possible (often required)
- Side effects are rare (unless frusemide or captopril is used)

Drawbacks of MAG3 renography
- Exposes patient to radiation
- Length of study (can take up to 1 hour)
- Prone to artifactual errors (e.g., due to renal impairment, posture, bladder effect, etc.)
- Limited anatomical information
- Equivocal results require a repeat procedure (usually F-15 study)
- Inaccurate outlining of ROIs can affect curve dynamics

(b) DMSA RENOGRAPHY

Overview
- ^{99m}Tc-DMSA has a high affinity for the renal cortex
- ^{99m}Tc-DMSA is the preferred radiopharmaceutical for static parenchymal imaging
- Provides the most accurate assessment of relative renal function compared to other tracers

Following tracer injection, ^{99m}Tc-DMSA is mostly plasma protein bound, and therefore clearance by GFR is minimal. In the kidney, the cells of the proximal convoluted tubules (and the distal tubules to a lesser extent) extract the ^{99m}Tc-DMSA by tubular secretion allowing slow concentration of radioactivity in the renal cortex. After 3 hours, about 50% of the injected tracer is concentrated in the kidneys, remaining there for up to 24 hours. The majority of the other 50% is excreted unchanged in urine. Increased hepatic accumulation, and subsequent biliary excretion is noted in patients in renal failure. Owing to the slow renal extraction of ^{99m}Tc-DMSA, the optimal time for imaging is between 2 and 4 hours after tracer injection.

^{99m}Tc-DMSA scanning represents functioning tubular mass, yields excellent cortical images, and is an invaluable tool in the assessment of both adults and children.

Indications
- Assessment of relative renal function
- Detection of renal scarring with a sensitivity of 96% and specificity of 98% (due to urinary tract infections or reflux nephropathy in children)
- Investigation of renal anomalies (e.g., horseshoe, solitary, or ectopic kidneys)
- Examination of space occupying renal lesions

Technique and radiation
The optimal time for DMSA scanning remains an unresolved issue. Many units perform the study in the acute phase (i.e., during or soon after a UTI) in order to determine the extent of parenchymal involvement. Critics of such practice point out that an acute abnormality does not necessarily represent a permanent scar and a repeat scan is often required after 3–6 months to determine longstanding injury. Deferring the DMSA scan for such a period of time may avoid the initial examination.

^{99m}Tc-DMSA has no specific contraindication and no specific patient preparation is required, since uptake is independent of the hydration state

- A typical adult dose of 80–100 MBq (1 MBq/kg body weight) is injected into a peripheral vein
- Images are acquired after 2–6 hours (usually after 3 h). Imaging must be avoided within the first hour due to the presence of free ^{99m}Tc in urine
- Regions of interest are created around both kidneys as well as a background area between the kidneys. Subtraction of the background area count from the overall kidney count will result in the correct kidney count

To maximize the detection of scarring, various projections should be utilized to image the kidney. Posterior, right, and left posterior views are standard, but anterior views must be included if a pelvic or horseshoe kidney is suspected. Furthermore, in asymmetric kidneys (e.g., ectopic kidneys, scoliosis), anterior views must be obtained and split function expressed as a geometric mean of radioactivity in both posterior and anterior images.

Reports in literature have suggested that the use of single photon emission computed tomography (SPECT) resolution in the DMSA scan improves sensitivity in the detection of renal scarring, compared to planar imaging. While no guidelines exist at present, SPECT usage is primarily dependent on locally available technology.

A typical dose of 80 MBq for DMSA renography corresponds to an effective radiation dose of 1 mSv (equivalent to 6 months of background radiation).

Interpretation

Normal kidneys should have a homogenous parenchymal distribution with visible demarcation between the cortex and medulla. Preservation of cortical thickness is indicative of acute changes, while cortical thinning is in keeping with chronic damage. The size, shape, and location (normal or ectopic) of the kidneys is readily demonstrated. Scars or other deformities are seen as areas of decreased or absent activity within the parenchyma. Artifacts may arise in kidneys with congenital fetal lobulations or due to splenic overlapping of the left kidney.

Urinary tract infection

In the acute setting, DMSA may demonstrate a single wedge-shaped area or multiple areas of decreased or absent tracer activity. Some UTI may resolve without scar formation while scarring (single or multiple) may be the long-term sequalae in others. Scar formation is also associated with decreasing relative function in the ipsilateral side. In patients with complete dupplex upper tract, it is the lower moiety that is prone to reflux, and therefore more likely to demonstrate reflux-related scarring.

Renal anomalies
Functioning ectopic kidneys, usually found in the midline pelvic position, are easily visible due to increased tracer activity. A DMSA will also reveal horseshoe kidneys and confirm the presence of a functioning isthmus.

Renal masses
Renal masses (e.g., tumors or cysts) appear as either well-circumscribed or ill-defined areas of non-functioning kidney. Although DMSA scanning is not routinely utilized for the investigation of such lesions, it is useful in planning nephron-sparing renal surgery for patients with tumor in a single kidney or those with bilateral tumors.

Advantages
- Provides excellent cortical images
- Accurate split renal function estimation
- Non-nephrotoxic
- No significant complications
- Allergic reactions are exceptionally rare

Drawbacks
- Involves radiation
- Does not allow dynamic assessment of renal excretion

(c) OBTAINING A GLOMERULAR FILTRATION RATE (GFR)

Overview
- GFR estimation is invaluable in the management of patients with or at risk of renal impairment
- GFR is defined as the volume of blood from which a solute is cleared by glomerular filtration through the Bowman's capsule per unit time (mL/min)
- GFR is regarded as a measure of global function
- Various techniques of GFR calculation have been described
- The more accurate techniques (e.g., inulin clearance) are impractical for routine medical use, but the more workable

methods (e.g., serum creatinine, 24-urine for creatinine clearance) are prone to inaccuracies
- Radionuclide techniques for GFR estimation can be utilized

The ideal radioactive tracer for this purpose would have the following properties:

- Be cleared solely, completely, and unmodified by glomerular filtration
- Should not undergo tubular secretion or resorption. Any tubular secretion will increase the resultant GFR value
- Be non-toxic, stable, and not bound to serum proteins
- Be readily measured in blood or urine
- Should have a constant clearance irrespective of plasma concentration

While inulin fulfils all criteria, it is impractical for clinical use. The chelating agents ^{99m}Tc DTPA and ^{51Cr} EDTA, which have a similar clearance to inulin, are therefore utilized. This method assumes that following injection, the tracer is equally distributed between the intravascular and extracellular fluid compartment after 2 hours, and the removal of a small but constant proportion by the kidneys will result in a proportional drop in tracer concentration in the blood. Decreasing tracer concentration can be estimated by taking serial venous blood samples at clearly defined intervals post tracer injection. Plotting the log of plasma tracer concentration over time will enable GFR estimation.

Indications
This technique can be used if employment of other techniques are impractical (e.g., if 24-hour urine collection is difficult, or if a high muscle mass might distort creatinine-based tests). General indications for GFR estimation include—

- Any clinical situation requiring an accurate measurement of absolute renal function
- Follow-up in patients with chronic renal disease
- Prior to administration of nephrotoxic therapy (e.g., chemotherapy)

Technique and radiation
No specific patient preparation is required, but ensure that the patient is well hydrated and empties the bladder prior to injection. For GFR studies:

- Doses used are 10 MBq for [99mTc] DTPA and 3 MBq for [51Cr] EDTA
- A pre-tracer injection venous blood sample is taken for background activity
- The tracer is injected and the exact time noted
- A heparinized blood sample is taken at 90, 150, 210, 270 minutes following injection and corrected (minus background activity) plasma tracer concentration can be plotted against time. Studies have shown that a minimum of four blood samples are required for accurate results
- Plotting the log of tracer concentration will result in a linear curve. Extrapolation of this line back to time zero will indicate the effective volume of distribution. The GFR is then calculated as the product of the distribution volume and the slope of the linear log curve, using the formula

$$GFR = V \lambda$$

where λ is the slope and V is injected tracer dose/distribution dose (see fig 4.3).

The *Gates* technique for GFR estimation, though not in common use, involves analysis of tracer activity in the kidneys between the 2- and 3-minute intervals following tracer injection. While the obvious advantage of this technique is the speed of the test and the absence of blood tests, its accuracy has been doubted. This technique has therefore fallen out of favor and most centers use a serial venous sampling method.

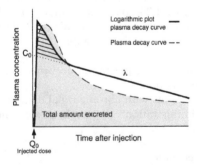

FIGURE 4.3. Logarithmic plot of plasma decay curve in single injection clearance techniques (with permission from *Comprehensive Urology*, Weiss, Mosby, 2001, 137)

An alternative to blood sampling is using three urine samples over 3 hours to measure urinary tracer concentration, but difficulties and inaccuracies in specimen collection make this method unattractive.

A typical dose of 10 MBq for ^{99m}Tc DTPA and 3 MBq for ^{51Cr} for EDTA for GFR studies corresponds to reasonably small effective radiation doses of 0.1 mSv and 0.007 mSv, respectively. It is therefore feasible to perform serial studies safely if clinically indicated.

Interpretation

Although cumbersome, these single injection filtration markers techniques provide a more accurate GFR reading than that obtained with traditional creatinine based methods. The GFR value obtained may be used uncorrected to evaluate changes in renal function for an individual patient. However, since GFR varies with age, gender, and body mass, it is recommended that a normalized GFR based on the standard body surface area of 1.73 m^2 be used for comparisons.

- Normal values are 130 mL/min/1.73 m^2 (men) and 120 mL/min/ 1.73 m^2 (women) with a variation coefficient of 14–18%
- Normalized GFR for the newborn is almost half that of the adult, with a gradual increase to adult values by the age 2
- GFR declines by roughly 1% per year after age 40
- Other factors affecting the GFR are time of day (10% higher in the afternoon than at midnight); pregnancy (up to 50% higher in the first trimester); high protein meal (gradual rise in GFR within an hour), and exercise (a transient reduction occurs)

Advantages
- Accurate
- No need for 24-hour urine collections
- Mandatory in clinical trials investigating progressive renal failure

Drawbacks
- Invasive—repeated blood samples
- Involves a small amount of radiation
- Lengthy procedure
- Artifacts can be caused by inaccurate recording of times, tracer extravasation at injection site, significant edema, or ascites (due to altered body compartment distribution)

(d) BONE SCAN

Overview
- Bone scintigraphy is the most commonly performed nuclear medicine study
- Diagnostic accuracy of about 95% for skeletal metastatic disease
- Invaluable tool in the staging of urological cancers
- Primary urological malignancies (prostate and kidney) are a common cause of skeletal secondaries

The information provided by the bone scan reflects metabolic activity within the bones. The most commonly used disphosphonate tracer, 99m Tc-methylenediphosphonate (medronate), is adsorbed onto the surface of bone crystals. The exact mechanism of this high phosphate uptake is unclear, but it reflects osteoblastic activity and skeletal vascularity at sites of active bone formation. Given its ability to detect the functional and metabolic response of bone to disease, the bone scan will often be positive even before plain X-ray changes are apparent. Bone scan findings are often non-specific and clues can be derived from the spatial distribution of activity throughout the skeleton and correlation with plain radiographic images. Serum markers of bone metabolic activity can prove useful and in rare instances a bone biopsy may be required to clarify the nature of a bone scan abnormality.

Indications
Although a number of other non-urological indications exist, the principal reasons for its use in the urological patient include—

- Staging of cancer (mainly prostate and kidney)
- Assessment of response to therapy in patients with cancer (e.g., prostate)
- Investigation of bone pain in urological patients
- Investigation of hypercalcemia

Technique and radiation
Medronate is a stable phosphate analog, with more than 50% of the administered activity concentrating in the bone and the rest rapidly cleared by the kidneys (by glomerular filtration). This allows good contrast between bone and soft tissue. The regional skeletal calcium content does not influence tracer uptake in bone. In addition, patients on oral bisphosphonate therapy do

not need to stop their medication as typical doses used in oral therapy do not affect medronate metabolism. However, intravenous treatment using large doses (e.g., for hypercalcemia) may temporarily reduce tracer uptake by normal bone and in such cases although bony metastases may still be visualized, it is recommended that bone scan be deferred for 4 weeks after completion of intravenous bisphosphonate therapy.

No specific contraindications exist.

- The typical dose of 500 MBq may have to be increased for SPECT or pinhole (for small bones) imaging, and in patients unable to remain still for long enough. SPECT improves lesion detection rate and provides improved resolution images
- Patients are required to be well hydrated (500 mL of clear fluid between injection and imaging)
- Patients must also be instructed to void several times to decrease bladder radiation and residual urine volume which may obscure the sacral bone
- Although a three-phase study (arterial, blood pool, delayed static imaging) is performed for the detection of inflammatory conditions, this is rarely required in urological patients
- Maximal bone uptake occurs after 2 hours, so delayed static whole body imaging is typically performed after 3–4 hours. Longer intervals (6 h) are used for older and obese patients and those in renal failure
- Whole body images can be taken from a variety of angles and spot images of a specific area of interest are also useful. Image density can be affected by distance from the camera and malpositioning of the patient must be avoided

A typical dose of 500 MBq for bone scan corresponds to an effective radiation dose of 4.5 mSv (equivalent to 27 months of background radiation).

Interpretation

Factors affecting bone scan
A number of benign and malignant bone disorders may result in positive findings on the bone scan. Fractures, infections, necrosis, Paget's disease, degenerative changes and primary bone tumors are common causes. Other flaws may arise as a result of—

- Pronounced lumbar lordosis or scoliosis and may result in seemingly asymmetrical uptake

- Residual tracer in the urinary tract which may obscure skeletal areas of interest (consider catheterising the patient)
- Excessive patient movement during imaging
- Extravasation or spillage of tracer which may confuse analysis (remove/change clothing if required)

The normal bone scan

Assessment of the bone scan requires careful examination not only of the skeleton, but also the soft tissue and renal tract as a number of other incidental non-skeletal abnormalities may be found. In the normal adult—

- There is symmetrical uptake about the spine, with a virtual mirror image between the left and right hemi-skeleton
- There should be uniform uptake throughout the skeleton, although there is greater activity in sites of high metabolic activity, such as joint margins, weight-bearing areas, and points of muscle insertion

In children and adolescents, there is increased uptake at the epiphyseal growth areas.

Soft tissue like the urinary tract is virtually always visualised under normal circumstances. The absence of renal visualisation may suggest a "superscan". The breast also often shows up in normal studies. Other organs may demonstrate increased uptake, often suggesting local pathological process (e.g., hydronephrosis).

The bone scan in skeletal metastatic disease

The majority of focal abnormalities, including bony metastases, appear as areas of increased tracer uptake (hotspots) (see Fig 4.4), but may in some instances be tracer poor. In general, a metastatic osteoblastic response is required for a positive hotspot on bone scan. For practical purposes, a negative result rules out the presence of metastatic disease, since false-negative results are rare. Although virtually any malignancy can spread to the bones, primary tumors in the prostate, breast, and lung are the common sources. Metastatic lesions are usually confined to the axial skeleton, but can sometimes affect the non-marrow-containing skeleton.

The bone scan in metastatic prostate cancer

- Roughly a third of patients with prostate cancer (CAP) will present with skeletal metastases

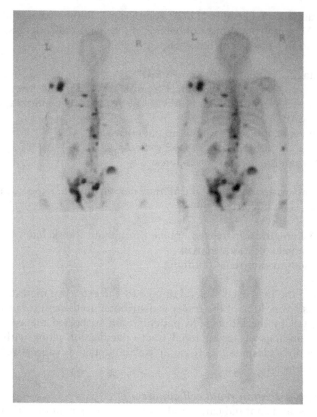

FIGURE 4.4. Bone scan showing widespread metastatic hotspots

- Typically, multiple sclerotic deposits are located in the pelvis and lumbar spine, although any part of the skeleton may be involved
- Skeletal spread is uncommon (<2%) in CAP patients with a PSA of <2 ng/mL and present in >90% of cases with a PSA >50 ng/mL
- Bone scans may also have a prognostic role in that mortality at 2 years in patients with and without a positive scan at presentation is 45% and 20%, respectively
- Endocrine treatment does influence bone scan results, with patients on hormonal manipulation for a period either demonstrating a negative bone scan (after being positive initially) or showing progression with appearance of new lesions

Though the precise role of bone scintigraphy in the management of CAP remains a subject of debate, the general indications specific to this disease include—

1. Staging patients with known CAP
2. Before embarking on radical treatment (even if PSA low)
3. In patients with a high PSA without histological confirmation of CAP
4. Increase in PSA in follow-up patients with CAP
5. New onset bone pain in CAP patients
6. To monitor treatment response

Patients with disseminated CAP may demonstrate a "superscan", which is characterized by—

• A symmetrical increased uptake throughout the skeleton
• Minimal soft tissue activity
• Absent or dim renal outlining

Due to the increased skeletal uptake by the extensive metastatic disease, very little of the tracer is distributed to the soft tissue or excreted by the kidneys. In patients with suspected metastatic CAP, findings of absent renal tract opacification along with a generally widespread increase in skeletal uptake is suggestive of a "superscan".

The bone scan in renal cell cancer
Bone scan is not indicated in the routine assessment of patients with kidney cancer since metastatic spread is uncommon in organ confined tumors. There is little evidence to advocate its routine use prior to radical surgery. In patients with skeletal involvement, the lesions often appear as large areas with a tracer-poor center surrounded by a rim of tracer activity. In some instances, these deposits may be completely photon deficient and another radiological technique (e.g., MR scanning) should be performed if clinical suspicion persists.

Bone scan following therapy for tumors
Bone scans are often performed in order to assess response to treatment. A favorable response following chemotherapy, hormonal manipulation, or radiotherapy will slow tumor progression and may also permit repair of bone affected by metastatic disease. In such cases, bone scan performed in patients with known bony metastases within 3–6 months of treatment will

usually be positive but may revert to being normal once osteoblastic bone repair is complete. It is worth noting that this may not necessarily indicate a favorable response to treatment, as the bone scan does not represent the primary tumor or any other coexisting non-skeletal metastatic spread.

Bone scan versus other imaging techniques

Although plain X-ray correlation is often suggested in indeterminate bone scan findings, it must be remembered that both imaging techniques assess different parameters. A plain radiograph is primarily dependent on the amount of calcification present in a lesion, while bone scintigraphy is a measure of local bone vascularity. Sclerotic activity may be readily demonstrated by plain X-ray, but in osteolytic lesion up to half of trabecular bone may have to be lost before becoming obvious on plain imaging. In addition, lesions smaller than 1 cm in diameter may be missed on plain X-ray, but are readily visible on bone scan.

MR scanning has a diagnostic accuracy approaching that of bone scintigraphy in the detection of skeletal metastases. Its other advantages are the lack of radiation and its ability to help discriminate between malignant and benign collapse of vertebral bodies and also reveal coexisting spinal cord compression. Bone scan, however, is more readily available and allows rapid assessment of the whole skeleton.

Advantages
- Accurate method of bone metastases detection
- Whole skeleton imaged at once

Drawbacks
- Requires radiation
- Lengthy procedure
- Low specificity for skeletal metastases
- Prone to artifacts

(e) POSITRON EMISSION TOMOGRAPHY (PET) SCAN

Overview

In nuclear medicine studies, the planar imaging commonly utilized provides a tracer distribution image in two dimensions. The basic aim of PET scanning is to create an image representing three-dimensional (3D) distribution of tracer, by combining the use of positron-emitting radionuclides and emission CT. Initially, a research tool for a number of years, PET scanning is now emerging as a useful clinical tool in the management of patients with a variety of pathological conditions, although its efficacy for the urological patient is still undetermined.

Certain radioisotopes decay by releasing positrons, which are positively charged electrons. These positrons travel short distances (less than 2.5 mm) and collide with other electrons, which results in the release of two high-energy (511 keV) photons emitted at 180° to each other. The PET scanner comprises several rings of multiple crystal detectors which detect the emitted photon, thereby reconstructing a 3D image of tracer distribution within the body.

One of the advantages of PET scanning is that it utilizes isotopes of elements ubiquitous in the human body and therefore is able to image physiologically important chemicals throughout the body, providing useful functional and metabolic information. Nevertheless, the majority of these have a very short half-life and are impractical for routine clinical use and mainly confined to the research laboratory. Half-lives of ^{15}O, ^{13}N, and ^{11}C are 2, 10, and 20 minutes, respectively.

The mainstay of clinical PET scanning is ^{18}fluorine (half-life 2 h) which is used to produce ^{18}fluorine-2-D-deoxyglucose (^{18}FDG), an analog of glucose. FDG, like glucose, is preferentially transported in tumor cells via specific glucose transporters, due to their inherently increased rate of metabolism and glycolysis. Once within the cell, FDG undergoes phosphorylation by hexokinase to form FDG-6-phosphate, following which it becomes inert and takes no further part in glycolytic pathway. It remains trapped in the tumor cell, and subsequent accumulation will eventually increase tracer activity to levels detectable by the PET scanner. The tracer is excreted through the kidneys. Because small amounts of tracer can be visualized, early tumor detection is possible even before other cross-sectional imaging (like CT or MRI) can detect structural changes. Other tracers, apart from FDG, continue to be developed and tested but remain some way off from entering the clinical setting.

A dedicated full ring PET scanner is the gold standard, but it is expensive. An acceptable alternative is to use a modified multi-head gamma camera. This has the advantage in that it is cheaper and can be used for SPECT imaging. Though costly, a dedicated PET scanner is quicker, more sensitive, has superior resolution compared to the gamma camera, and does not require a collimator. Combining a CT scanner and PET scanner within a single imaging scaffold will provide excellent anatomical as well as functional information and is likely to become the PET imaging technique of the future.

The majority of data on PET scanning arises from studies in brain metabolism and non-urological cancers (e.g., lung, colorectal, head and neck, lymphoma). At present clear guidelines for the use of PET in the management of urological patients do not exist and clinical practice is based on local availability and physician preference. Data assessing PET performance in urological malignancies remains sparse and occasionally conflicting, although further evidence may confirm an emerging role.

Indications
The non-urological indications are not discussed here. Currently, though there are no absolute urological indications, PET may contribute in the following pathological processes:

- Testicular tumors
  - Primary tumor staging
  - Early detection of recurrent disease
  - Assessment of residual tumor burden after therapy
- Renal cell cancer
  - Initial staging of local and distant disease
  - Detection of recurrence
- Bladder cancer
  - Detection of recurrent disease (if other imaging ambivalent)
- Detection of bony metastases (if bone scan equivocal)

Technique and radiation
The are no specific contraindications to PET scanning except for women who are pregnant and breastfeeding.

Patient preparation
- Patients advised to avoid food for 4–6 hours and oral intake restricted to non-sugary clear fluid
- Blood glucose estimation is performed just prior to the examination to ensure low glucose levels (high levels inhibit FDG uptake by cells)
- In addition, buscopan (20 mg) and/or diazepam may be administered to reduce FDG uptake by the intestines and muscles, respectively

- A preliminary background scan is performed before up to 400 MBq of FDG is injected intravenously
- Imaging is performed between 45 and 90 minutes after tracer injection
- A whole body scan can be performed or imaging restricted to the area of interest, with or without simultaneous CT scanning

A maximal injected dose of 400 MBq corresponds to an effective radiation dose of 10 mSv (equivalent to up to 6 years of background radiation).

Interpretation

Since FDG-PET is a function of glucose metabolism, any organ with a higher metabolic rate will demonstrate greater tracer activity under normal circumstances (e.g., brain, intestines, liver, heart, etc.). Tracer uptake by malignant lesions will also depend on the rate of glycolysis. Although most tumors will demonstrate an inherently higher metabolic rate, some tumors (e.g., prostatic cancers) may have decreased proliferative activity and therefore not be apparent on PET images. The lower limit of the size of lesion detectable by PET scanning is 5 mm in diameter but is likely to improve in the future with improved resolution scanners.

Testicular tumors

Results of PET in the management of testicular tumors show the most promise compared to other renal tract cancers.

- *Primary disease*: PET has a superior performance profile than conventional imaging. CT scan has been reported to have false-negative and false-positive rates of as high as 59% and 25%, respectively, in low-stage disease. By contrast, a number of studies have demonstrated a higher specificity (87–100%), higher sensitivity (70–100%), and better negative predictive value for PET compared to CT scanning. If metastatic disease at presentation is obvious after conventional imaging, then PET has a rather limited role. It may, however, be of value in the assessment of patients with stage II disease and could potentially alter management. Furthermore, emerging evidence may suggest a role for PET in predicting response to chemotherapy, but more data is required

- *Recurrent disease*: patients presenting with raised tumor markers following previous therapy can represent a diagnostic dilemma, especially if conventional imaging is negative. PET scan performs better than CT in this instance and is more likely to detect recurrent disease earlier than CT or MRI. Some authors have advocated the use of PET as first line investigation in patients with suspected recurrence

- *Residual tumor*: PET can play a significant role in the treatment of patients with residual mass following radiotherapy or chemotherapy for seminoma. CT cannot confidently discriminate between malignant and fibrotic/necrotic tissue in up to 50% of cases. The positive predictive value of PET in such patients is between 80% and 96%. A negative PET scan is indicative of non-cancerous tissue in 88–90% of cases. Thus it is in this category of patients that PET has been found to be most useful

Renal cell cancer (RCC)
- *Primary disease*: even though the normal kidney will demonstrate FDG uptake, PET performs as well as CT in the characterization of a renal lesion as benign or malignant. Some renal cell cancers may be PET negative and therefore may be missed. Overall, PET is more likely to detect unsuspected metastatic disease compared to CT and this may hugely influence treatment options. Nevertheless, PET is not routinely indicated prior to radical nephrectomy at present

- *Recurrent disease*: PET can confidently distinguish between malignant and benign disease in patients with a previous history of RCC, presenting with a subsequent indeterminate lesion, in 75–100% of cases. Lymph node involvement and local or distant spread can be effectively identified by PET

Bladder cancer
Because of the urinary excretion of FDG, visualization of the bladder is difficult, and PET is not currently indicated in local staging of bladder cancer. Accuracy of lymph node detection is marginally better than with CT or MRI scan and further work is required in this subset of patients.

Prostate cancer
Slow glycolytic rates (resulting in poor FDG uptake), low-volume tumors, and suboptimal visualization of the prostate area (due to tracer accumulation in the bladder) have meant that PET has a rather limited role in investigating localized prostate cancer. It may, however, be useful in the detection of metastatic lymph

nodes, recurrent distant disease, and to monitor treatment response (e.g., to androgen deprivation). Emerging new tracers, including ^{11}C-methionine (amino acid tracer), ^{11}C-choline, and ^{11}C-acetate (both lipid based tracers) have shown promising results compared to FDG, but sparse data and their relatively short half-lives have made routine clinical use difficult.

PET is inferior to conventional bone scintigraphy in the detection of skeletal metastases but can be used to provide additional information if the latter is equivocal.

Advantages
- Uses biologically important radionuclides to provide pertinent functional and metabolic information
- Proven efficacy in other non-urological cancers
- Generally high specificity for malignant disease
- Whole body can be imaged at once
- Spatial resolution of 5 mm
- Can be combined with simultaneous CT to improve image resolution

Drawbacks
- Involves radiation
- Length of procedure
- Expensive (cost of collimator, scanner, and radiochemistry facility is high)
- Radionuclides with a short half-life may need to be produced on site
- Lack of anatomical landmarks (especially in the thorax and abdomen)
- Urinary excretion limits detection of bladder and prostate malignancies

Chapter 5
Urodynamics

(a) FREQUENCY VOLUME CHARTS

Overview
- Frequency volume charts (FVC) or voiding diaries are an extremely useful, non-invasive means of investigating the male and female urinary tracts
- All patients with troublesome lower urinary tract symptoms (LUTS) should complete an FVC as part of their initial management
- FVC allows a more objective baseline definition of the severity of the symptoms
- Useful for monitoring progress following therapy by providing feedback for both patient and physician

Indications
- Assessment of patients with LUTS
- Prior to urodynamic investigations
- Monitoring of patients with LUTS, especially pre- and post-treatment (medical, surgical, or bladder retraining drills)
- Patients with suspected nocturnal polyuria

Technique
- Minimum data collection period is 3 consecutive days, although 7 days is ideal
- The period of data collection should reflect the patient's usual routine (i.e., work day rather than a day off; or a combination of both)
- Patient must be instructed to void as normal

Standard practice is to ask the patient to complete the FVC prior to a urologist appointment, as this can be analyzed as part of the initial examination. The patient is instructed to accurately record their voiding pattern, including the following parameters:

- Mandatory —time of voids (including nighttime voids)
  —volume of each void
  —number of incontinent episodes
- Additional —times and volume of fluid intake (can become tedious)
  —record the presence and degree of urgency
  —use and number of incontinence pads

Interpretation
- Maximum voided volume is indicative of the maximal volumetric capacity of the bladder
- Average maximal voided volumes represent the functional capacity
- Daytime frequency of 3–4 hours is considered normal
- Degree of nocturia is usually dependent on the age of the patient

In adults, generally—
- Diurnal frequency is 5–7 voids
- Nocturnal frequency 0–1 void
- Normal voided volumes between 300 and 500 mL for women and 400 and 600 mL for men
- It is not unusual for the patients in their 50s and 60s to void once during the night and those in their 70s and 80s to have to get up 2 or 3 times nightly

Distinct patterns can be noted on FVC analysis:
- Normal volumes and normal frequency
- Normal volumes, but increased frequency: polyuria may be due to increased fluid intake, diabetes insipidus or mellitus
- Decreased volume: small volume voids both day and night might suggest detrusor overactivity (variable volumes) or bladder inflammation, sensory urgency or carcinoma in situ (fixed reduced volumes)
- Normal early morning void followed by decreased variable volumes for the rest of the day: usually due to a non-organic cause
- Increased nighttime frequency: nocturnal polyuria exists if >30% of total daily urine is passed at night time and may be idiopathic or secondary to congestive cardiac failure or renal failure

Bladder outflow obstruction (BOO):
- There are no typical FVC patterns that characterize BOO

- A range of features can be noted including small volume voids, frequency, nocturia, and urgency

Detrusor overactivity:
- A common finding is a pattern of frequent voids during the day and night with variable volumes
- Often episodes of marked urgency and urge incontinence depending on the symptom severity
- Important to exclude other possible causes of such irritative symptoms including an intravesical mass lesion or CIS (cystoscopy is mandatory in patients over 40 years of age)
- An important feature is the fixed nature of the reduced void volumes (functional capacity) accompanying the frequency

Psychogenic pattern:
- Psychological difficulties often affect the bladder
- Patterns are difficult to predict
- Certain features, in the absence of any significant bladder pathology, are suggestive of a non-organic etiology for LUTS. These include—
  - Variable symptoms (worse during periods of stress and improve in between times)
  - Absent nocturia but marked daytime symptoms
  - Large first morning void, but small variable voids subsequently through the day

Patients who undergo bladder retraining must complete regular FVC in order to provide important biofeedback for the patient.

- FVC is a simple and non-invasive tool which is often underutilized
- Well accepted by patients
- A minimum of 3 days' data is required
- Limitations include
  - A minority fail to complete the diary due to a variety of reasons
  - Accuracy in record-keeping is important for pertinent data analysis
  - Symptoms may vary from period to period even within the same patient and it is important to avoid over-interpretation, but to use it as an adjunct to urodynamic assessment

(b) FLOW RATE STUDY

Overview
- Simplest and often the most useful of urodynamic techniques
- Measures the volume of urine voided per unit time (mL/s)
- Inherently inferior to pressure-flow studies in the assessment of voiding difficulties
- Provides useful and practical data to direct initial management

Urine flow rate (FR) or uroflowmetry is—

- Primarily determined by outflow resistance and detrusor function, and an abnormal flow rate may be secondary to dysfunction in either
- Altered by abdominal straining and therefore only provides a measure of total voiding function
- Mandatory in virtually all males, and some female urological patients
- Often the only investigation required in >60% of men with uncomplicated bladder outflow obstruction (BOO)

A basic understanding of standard nomenclature is required.

- Flow pattern can be described as continuous or interrupted
- Voided volume (VV) is the total volume of urine expelled
- Maximum flow rate (Q_{max}) denotes the maximum measured value of the flow rate
- Flow time indicates the time over which the flow occurred
- Time to maximum flow is the time taken from commencement of flow to reach Q_{max}
- Average flow rate (Q_{ave}) can be calculated dividing the voided volume by the flow time

Indications
- Males
  - With symptoms suggestive of bladder outflow obstruction
  - Recurrent UTI
  - Before and following surgery on the lower urinary tract

- Females
  - Symptoms suggesting outlet obstruction
  - Recurrent UTI

- Prior to surgery for stress incontinence (to establish satisfactory detrusor function)

• Children
  - Assessment of dysfunctional voiding

Technique
• Should be performed when the patient's bladder is adequately filled and there is a normal desire to void
• Ideally, patients ought to have completed a FVC prior to flow tests
• Patients are asked to drink at least a liter of fluid at home prior to attending hospital. In addition, intra-test hydration is maintained by asking patients to drink a further liter of water during the test. Flow rates following a catheter fill are less physiological than free flow rates
• Due to the variability in FR traces, the patient is asked to perform three flow rates, each of a voided volume similar to those on the frequency volume chart
• Voiding should occur in privacy, with male patients standing up and females voiding sitting down on a commode
• In adults, a minimal voided volume of 150 mL is required to allow meaningful analysis of the FR trace, while a voided volume of >600 mL may result in erroneous results secondary to bladder overdistension and detrusor decompensation. In such cases the uroflowmetry must be repeated. Patients with repeated voids less than 150 mL are likely to have bladder outflow obstruction in about 70% of cases, if pressure-flow tests are performed
• Ultrasound estimation of bladder residual volume must be performed following micturition to measure residual urine volume

Most electronic uroflowmeters provide a paper tracer (paper speed 0.25 cm/s), which can be kept with the patient records for comparison at a later stage. Uroflowmeters usually have an accuracy of >95% and use a variety of principles in order to calculate flow rates, including—

1. Rotating disk method: urine falls onto a disk spinning at a constant speed. Urine slows down the speed of rotation. The power required by the motor to keep the disk spinning at a constant speed is proportional to the flow rate
2. Electronic dipstick (capacitance) method: urine collects in a chamber mounted with a dipstick capacitor. The change in

capacitance due to urine in the chamber is indicative of the flow rate
3. Gravimetric method: this simply involves the calculation of urine flow rate by measuring the weight of voided urine

Interpretation

Normal (see Fig 5.1a)
Assuming a reasonable voided volume, the flow pattern, Q_{max}, and Q_{ave} are the most reliable and most commonly used parameters. Normal values vary with patient gender, age, and voided volumes. The most physiologically accurate traces are derived with voided volumes of between 200 and 500 mL. The normal flow rate—

- Is usually a bell-shaped, continuous pattern with a sharp take-off and a reasonably rapid final phase descent
- The Q_{max} should be reached within the first 5 seconds of the flow rate (or within the first 30% of the trace)
- Young men (<40 years of age) usually have a Q_{max} of over 25 mL/s, which decreases with age to over 15 mL/s in men over the age of 60 years
- Women generally have higher flow rates than men (20–40 mL/s) with a less significant age-related decline

Flow patterns
Examination of the flow patterns may provide sufficient indication of the underlying pathology. The flow may be continuous or interrupted. Interrupted flow patterns only come in a few varieties due to the following causes:

- Straining: traces from patients increasing their intra-abdominal pressure while voiding, either because of BOO or an underactive detrusor, will demonstrate a slow, irregular, multi-peaked pattern. The flow may be continuous (usually with each void) or interrupted (poorly sustained or insufficient detrusor contractions). Pressure-flow studies are the next step

- Detrusor–sphincter dyssynergia (DSD): the lack of coordination between detrusor contractions and urethral sphincter relaxation when voiding, in patients with neurological abnormalities or extreme anxiety, can result in asymmetrical and interrupted traces. In general, these patients will have a greater Q_{max} than those seen during straining

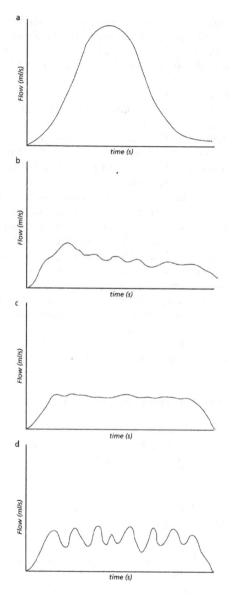

FIGURE 5.1. Flow rate patterns—(**a**) normal, (**b**) bladder outflow obstruction, (**c**) stricture pattern, (**d**) neuropathic detrusor–sphincter dyssynergia

- Artifacts: cruising (moving the urine stream when voiding into the funnel) and squeezing the tip of the penis when voiding can result in irregular flow patterns. Flow rates must be repeated in such patients after adequate instructions.

Maximum flow rate (Q_{max})

Care must be taken in the evaluation of maximum flow rates due to the absence of simultaneous pressure studies. However, in men in general, a Q_{max} of >15 mL/s is indicative of non-obstruction in 80% of patients, while over 70% of patients are truly obstructed with a Q_{max} of <10 mL/s. Given the effect of both detrusor contractility and outlet obstruction of the flow rate, the Q_{max} may be decreased in a variety of conditions, including BOO, urethral strictures, hypotonic detrusor, abdominal straining, and DSD. Detrusor overactivity may result in an increased Q_{max} due to the high contraction velocities ("fast bladder"). A number of normograms exist to help categorize Q_{max} at various voided volumes into the obstructed or normal range.

Women, as a result of a shorter urethra will demonstrate higher Q_{max} values compared to their male counterparts. Women with genuine stress incontinence may also have faster flow rates due to decreased outlet resistance.

The following table denotes the minimal acceptable Q_{max} values for males and females based on age and voided volumes (Table 5.1).

Flow rates in specific conditions (see Fig 5.1b–d)

Bladder outflow obstruction
- The FR is characterized by a low Q_{max} (5–6 mL/s), decreased Q_{ave}, with the Q_{ave} greater than half of Q_{max}

TABLE 5.1. The minimal acceptable Q_{max} values for males and females based on age and voided volumes

Age (yr)	Min voided volume (mL)	Q_{max} (mL/s) males	Q_{max} (mL/s) females
4–7	100	10	10
8–13	100	12	15
14–45	200	21	18
46–65	200	12	15
66–80	200	9	10

- In addition, the flow time is prolonged, with a prolonged terminal phase (associated with dribbling)
- Usually, the pattern is that of sustained low flow with minimal variation
- Note that up to 20% of patients may demonstrate a "normal" Q_{max} as the outflow obstruction may be overcome by significant elevations in intravesical pressures

Urethral stricture
- Constrictive bladder outlet obstruction—a "plateau" trace is the norm
- There is a sharp uptake to reach Q_{max} within the first 3–5 seconds with a subsequent flat regular trace culminating in a sharp decline on completion of voiding
- There is little difference between Q_{max} and Q_{ave}

Detrusor overactivity
- Best demonstrated urodynamically by pressure-flow studies
- The relatively high end-filling intravesical pressure typically produces an exaggeration of normal flow with a higher than expected Q_{max}

Detrusor underactivity
- Usually produces a prolonged symmetrical curve with a reduced Q_{max}
- Typically, the time to reach Q_{max} is prolonged as well
- Some patients may exhibit a straining pattern in order to augment bladder emptying
- Ultimately pressure-flow studies are required for definitive diagnosis

---

- Uroflowmetry is cheap, fast, and non-invasive
- Indicated in virtually all men with LUTS
- Can identify patients requiring more extensive urodynamic evaluation
- Q_{max} of >15 mL/s suggests non-obstruction in most males
- Characteristic patterns often associated with common lower urinary tract pathologies
- Limitations include the lack of bladder pressure data, intra-patient variability, and the possibility of artifactual errors

(c) RESIDUAL BLADDER URINE VOLUME ESTIMATION

Overview
The post-voiding residual (PVR) urine is defined as the volume of fluid remaining in the bladder immediately following the completion of micturition and—

- Allows simple generalization about the urinary tract
- Should routinely follow after uroflowmetry
- Is an integral aspect of urodynamic evaluation and should follow the micturition phase of pressure-flow studies
- Provides data on interaction between detrusor activity and outlet obstruction
- Is prone to variations depending on patient surroundings, initial pre-micturition bladder volume and measuring techniques
- Repeated measurements improve validity

Indications
- Males and females
  - With any lower urinary tract symptoms
  - Follow-up of patients with acute or chronic urinary retention
  - Recurrent UTI
  - Abdominal or suprapubic pain
  - (Males) before and following bladder outlet surgery
  - (Females) before and following incontinence surgery

- Children
  - Assessment of dysfunctional voiding
  - Recurrent UTI

Technique
Testing under clinical situations can result in incomplete and artificially elevated PVR volumes. Sequential measurements are therefore advised. Methods to estimate PVR include—

a. Ultrasound (true volume often underestimated but most practical)
b. Instrumentation (catheter or cystoscope)
c. Radiography (IVU or videourodynamics)
d. Radioisotopes (gamma camera)

It is also important to record—

- The time from micturition to PVR estimation (the latter should ideally immediately follow the former, especially if the patient is undergoing a diuresis)
- Presence of any bladder diverticula (urine in a large diverticula may or may not be included in PVR estimation)

Occasionally in children, re-entry of refluxed urine back into the bladder following micturition may be confused with PVR.

Interpretation

Considerable debate exists as to the definition of a normal PVR volume.

- Generally, a PVR of <50 mL is regarded as normal in adults
- The absence of residual urine, though clinically useful, does not adequately exclude BOO or lower urinary tract dysfunction, as the intravesical pressure may be sufficient to overcome degrees of outlet obstruction
- Even small PVR volumes may be significant in symptomatic patients, especially those with recurrent infections and bladder calculus
- PVR of >200 mL is abnormal and regular USS surveillance of the bladder and kidneys is recommended due to the risk of upper tract obstruction
- PVR consistently >300 mL is in keeping with chronic retention and intervention may be advisable (unless this represents a low-pressure system in an asymptomatic patient)
- Consistently increased PVR volume is more likely to represent impaired detrusor contractility with or without coexistent BOO, rather than simply being a function of BOO in isolation. It is important to bear this in mind when managing patients with suspected BOO and therefore repeated measurements and correlation with pressure-flow studies are advised

---

(d) PRESSURE-FLOW CYSTOMETRY STUDIES

Overview

Cystometry is a urodynamic study of pressure-volume relationships of the bladder and urethra. The purpose of cystometric testing is to simulate the physiological mechanisms of lower urinary tract dysfunction, thereby enabling appropriate management.

The technique applied will affect overall results and standardization of the methodology is essential to enhance reproducibility and allow comparisons. Moreover, results must be interpreted in conjunction with the patient's symptoms and clinical picture.

- Simple filling cystometry assesses changes during the bladder filling and can evaluate parameters such as detrusor activity, bladder capacity, compliance, and abnormal bladder sensation
- Voiding cystometry (or pressure-flow cystometry) can synchronously measure intravesical pressure changes and urethral flow during micturition to determine the mechanism of abnormal voiding

Indications

Cystometry is time-consuming, invasive, can be uncomfortable and is not indicated in all patients presenting with symptoms. It is best avoided if the clinical picture is sufficient to make a satisfactory working diagnosis, especially if conservative therapeutic options are being considered. Other indications include—

- Severe irritative LUTS (especially if symptoms do not correlate with objective physical findings)
- Assessment of troublesome urinary incontinence (stress or urge) if etiology unclear
- Assessment of the neuropathic bladder
- Suspected bladder outflow obstruction (especially in males <50 years of age and associated irritative symptoms) (Fig. 5.2)
- If invasive surgery to the lower urinary tract is planned
- In treatment failure following therapy

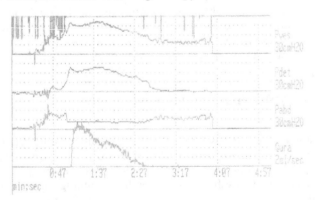

FIGURE 5.2. BOO—low flow (8 mL/s), high pressure (90 cmH$_2$0) (Courtesy of Mr C Betts, Hope Hospital, Salford)

Technique

Prior to cystometry, all patients must undergo—

- Full history and physical examination (including pelvic and neurological)
- Urine microscopy and culture
- Frequency volume chart analysis
- Uroflowmetry (in males)
- Estimation of the post-micturition residual urine volume

Subtraction cystometry is the gold standard, with simultaneous measurement of the intravesical (Pves) and intra-abdominal pressure (Pabd). The detrusor pressure (Pdet) is calculated by subtracting the intra-abdominal pressure from the intravesical pressure to eliminate the effects of straining. Some transducer catheters also allow concurrent urethral pressure measurement.

- Microtransducer catheters are more accurate but expensive and can produce artifacts
- Water- and air-filled balloon catheters are reasonably accurate, less expensive, and represent a realistic alternative

The transducers are calibrated and pressure monitoring occurs continuously till completion of the study. Although carbon dioxide cystometry can be used, in most instances liquid cystometry is performed with either water, normal saline, or contrast material infused into the bladder at room temperature. Liquid cystometry is more physiological and permits a voiding study.

Cystometry can be performed in the supine, sitting, or standing position, although the latter two are more physiological and therefore more desirable than the former.

- Following voluntary bladder emptying, a 6–10F single (infusion only), double- (simultaneous infusion and intravesical pressure measurement) or triple-lumen catheter (for infusion as well as bladder and urethral pressure measurement) is inserted into the bladder
- If a separate catheter is used for bladder filling, this must be removed before the voiding phase
- Record initial residual urine volume and bladder pressure
- A 2-mm diameter saline-filled catheter is placed in the rectum or vagina for assessment of intra-abdominal pressure

- The bladder should be filled on top of any existing residual, unless the patient normally self-catheterizes (in which case, the residual urine must be drained). Otherwise, removal of residual urine may significantly alter bladder function and behavior on urodynamics, especially affecting compliance, detrusor overactivity, and cystometric capacity
- Filling rate may be slow (<10 mL/min), medium (10–100 mL/min), or fast (greater than 100 mL/min). Most investigators use a medium-fill rate, although higher rates may be utilized to provoke detrusor overactivity in patients with marked urgency. Bladder compliance can be influenced by rate of filling and a low fill rate (10–20 mL/min) is advisable for neuropathic patients
- During filling, the following parameters are recorded:
  - Volume at first desire to void
  - Volume at normal desire to void
  - Volume at urgency
  - Maximum cystometric capacity (volume when patient unable to delay micturition)
  - Change in bladder compliance
  - Occurrence of involuntary detrusor contractions
- Provocative maneuvers, such as coughing, straining, walking in place, jumping, hand-washing, and listening to running water are helpful to demonstrate leakage and whether the leakage is related to uninhibited detrusor contractions or stress incontinence
- Once cystometric capacity is reached, the patient is brought up to the upright position (sitting or standing) and further provocative tests can be performed to estimate a Valsalva leak point pressure (abdominal pressure at which stress leakage occurs)
- The patient then voids into a uroflowmeter, and measurements are made of voiding pressures, voided volume, flow rate, and residual volume

Interpretation

Normal function

In the normal bladder, bladder pressures (Pdet and Pves) should remain low and constant during filling up to the point of voiding. Compliance (change in volume for a given change in pressure) remains high till cystometric capacity is reached. Prior to voiding, there is urethral sphincter relaxation, followed by a smooth, coordinated detrusor contraction resulting in a low-pressure, high-flow urine stream till the bladder is completely empty. The flow pattern in a pressure-flow study should be representative of free flow studies in the same patient.

Normal values for parameters measured during the filling phase are subject to considerable variation:

- First desire to void occurs at approximately 50% of capacity (150–250 mL)
- Normal desire to void occurs at approximately 75% of capacity (200–350 mL)
- Urgency may occur at approximately 90% of capacity (300–500 mL)
- Maximum cystometric capacity is 350–500 mL in women and 400–600 mL in men. This can be correlated with the maximum voided volume in the patient's frequency volume charts
- Pressure changes must remain small (Pdet <15 cmH$_2$O) and be without any undue sensation of urgency, up to the point of micturition
- If measured, the urethral pressure is seen to rise slightly during filling to aid continence

The detrusor contracts throughout voiding, preceded by external sphincteric relaxation.

- In males, voiding occurs with a Pdet of 35–50 cmH$_2$O with flow rates of between 15 and 30 mL/s depending on age
- Pdet in females remains low on voiding (10–40 cmH$_2$O) with a resulting flow rate of 30–35 mL/s

Common abnormalities on cystometry

Abnormal results do not necessarily indicate pathology as inconsistent values may occasionally be noted in normal, asymptomatic patients and are of little clinical significance. Abnormalities noted in symptomatic patients are more consequential. Some characteristic findings associated with common abnormalities are described below.

Filling cystometry
1. Detrusor overactivity (see Fig 5.3)
   - Characterized by phasic elevations of detrusor pressure over baseline during the filling phase, irrespective of the magnitude, which reproduce the patient's symptoms
   - Pressure rises may occur spontaneously or on provocation while the patient tries to inhibit micturition
   - Pressure rises are associated with urgency and may or may not be associated with urine leakage

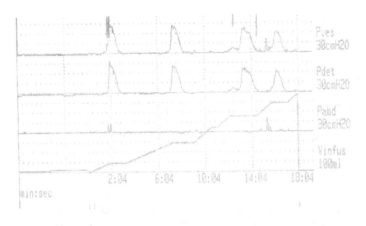

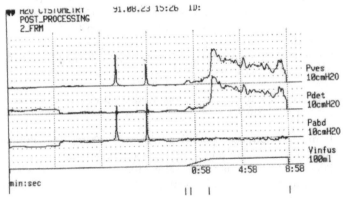

FIGURE 5.3. Urodynamics traces showing unstable detrusor contractions during filling cystometry (Courtesy of Mr C Betts, Hope Hospital, Salford)

- The severity of the condition may be assessed by the volume at which contractions occur, the amplitude and duration of contractions, associated symptoms, and whether the contraction resulted in leakage or a full void
- In neuropathic patients, overactive detrusor contractions are termed "neurogenic detrusor overactivity."

2. Loss of compliance
  - Reduced compliance illustrated by a steady rise in Pdet during filling is generally regarded as abnormal and poses a risk to the upper tracts

- Normal compliance has been calculated as a pressure rise of less than $1\,cmH_2O$ for every $37\,mL$ infused
- Compliance can be altered by infusion rate and volume as well as patient position
- Loss of compliance is noted in patients with a neuropathic bladder (e.g., secondary to cord injury or pelvic surgery), infection, interstitial cystitis, malignancy, fibrosis (e.g., after radiotherapy) and myelodysplasia

3. Sensory abnormalities
   - In sensory urgency there is urgency at low volumes and bladder capacity is reduced ($<250\,mL$) due to hypersensitivity, with no associated rise in Pdet
   - Pain on bladder filling is always abnormal
   - Reduced or absent sensation results in a large cystometric capacity with no real strong desire to void and is seen in neurologically abnormal patients

4. Genuine stress incontinence
   - Characterized by leakage that occurs with an increase in abdominal pressure without a rise in true detrusor pressure
   - The abdominal leak point pressure (Pabd at which stress leakage occurs) is used to determine the extent of stress leakage and correlates with sphincteric function
   - The higher the leak point pressure (LPP), the better the sphincteric function
   - Unlike the urethral pressure profile, the LPP reflects urethral function in the dynamic situation that produces incontinence and is more reliable than the urethral pressure profile for diagnosis of intrinsic sphincter deficiency
   - LPP of $<60\,cmH_2O$ represent intrinsic sphincter deficiency
   - In patients with stress incontinence, abdominal LPP $>100\,cmH_2O$ suggests urethral hypermobility as a causative factor

Voiding cystometry
1. Disorders of detrusor contractility
   - Except in the elderly population, a normal detrusor contraction will effect complete bladder emptying
   - The hypotonic or underactive detrusor is typified by contractions of inadequate magnitude and/or duration to effect complete bladder emptying, and a low flow rate in the absence of urethral obstruction
   - There are often associated rises in Pabd due to straining

- In the flaccid or acontractile bladder, no detrusor contractions are demonstrated during urodynamic studies
- Detrusor acontractility is often due to a neurological abnormality such as spinal cord injury or multiple sclerosis, but may also be idiopathic

2. Bladder outlet obstruction
   - Illustrated by a low flow rate associated with a high Pdet
   - The bladder may not empty completely
   - May be seen due to outlet overactivity (failure of sphincteric relaxation) or anatomical obstruction (e.g., prostatic hypertrophy or urethral stricture)
   - Generally, a Pdet higher than 60 cmH$_2$O with flow rate Q$_{max}$ of less than 10 mL/s implies obstruction in males
   - In females, a Pdet of >20 cmH$_2$O and Q$_{max}$ <15 mL/s is generally associated with obstruction
   - Given the varied nature of the pressure-flow relationship, various nomograms (e.g., International Continence Society [ICS], Schaefer and Spangberg nomograms) have been devised to assist making the diagnosis of obstruction. The ICS nomogram will categorize patients into three groups—unobstructed, obstructed and equivocal. The Schaefer (or LinPURR—linear passive urethral resistance relation) nomogram grades detrusor contractility and outlet obstruction. In addition, calculation of the Abrams–Griffiths number can help classify a pressure-flow study using the formula

   Abrams–Griffiths number = Pdet at Qmax − 2 × Q$_{max}$

   If the Abrams–Griffiths number is >40 the pressure-flow study is obstructed; if <20 the pressure-flow study is unobstructed. Otherwise the study is equivocal.

3. Detrusor–sphincter dyssynergia (DSD)
   - Lack of coordination between urethral relaxation and detrusor contraction in the neuropathic bladder results in spasms of involuntary sphincteric activity during attempted voiding
   - The end result is an intermittent flow pattern with a high fluctuating Pdet (rising as flow stops and falling as flow starts)
   - Such bladders rarely empty completely and high intravesical pressures can cause upper tract function deterioration

4. Dysfunctional voiding
   - A similar pattern to that seen in detrusor–sphincter dys-synergia, but the pattern is usually voluntary
   - Commonly seen in women and children who are anxious and due to sphincteric denervation in females following pelvic surgery

Limitations

Cystometry has a number of pitfalls:

- The artificial surroundings of the urodynamic laboratory can inhibit voiding in up to 30% of women
- Time-consuming, invasive, and prone to artifacts
- Lack of standardization of technical aspects, such as patient position, type of transducer/catheter, and filling rate may cause variable results
- A wide range of normal values; therefore not all abnormal results are significant
- Intra-patient variability on repeat examination
- Normal cystometric findings do not necessarily exclude a pathology

---

- Remains the most unequivocal method of assessing lower urinary tract function/dysfunction
- Indicated in patients with complex symptomatology and if surgery being considered
- Will readily demonstrate detrusor overactivity, compliance disorders, BOO, DSD, and incontinence
- Attention to technical detail is paramount
- Has recognized limitations

(e) URETHRAL PRESSURE PROFILE

Overview

Sufficient urethral pressure is mandatory for the maintenance of urinary incontinence. Urethral profile measurement (or urethral profilometry) is a technique used to record the intraluminal pressure changes within the entire length of the urethra. A satisfactory evaluation of urethral function can be made by a standard filling/voiding bladder urodynamic study, such that urethral closure mechanism is considered adequate if no incontinence is demonstrated and inadequate if there is obvious stress leakage. Demonstration of urinary stress leakage therefore represents a direct assessment of urinary incontinence, while urethral pressure profilometry (UPP) is a less direct method.

In clinical practice, because UPP has been plagued with inconsistencies and remains susceptible to artifactual errors, it offers little to patient management and does not enjoy widespread usage. The discussion in this chapter therefore will be limited to basic principles.

- Maximum urethral profile (MUP)—highest pressure recorded on the pressure profile
- Maximum urethral closure pressure (MUCP)—difference between the MUP and intravesical pressure
- Functional profile length (FPL)—length of urethra along which the urethral pressure exceeds intravesical pressure

Indications

As an isolated urodynamic test, UPP has little value and is not performed routinely in all centers. Possible indications include—

- Investigation of genuine urinary stress leakage
- Assessment of the urethra/bladder neck prior to surgery if urinary undiversion is being considered
- Assess the efficacy of sphincterotomy in patient with neurogenic bladder dysfunction
- Assessment of post-prostatectomy incontinence

Technique

UPP measurement is contraindicated in the presence of a urinary tract infection. Some centers give a single dose of prophylactic antibiotics prior to the test. UPP measurement may be made—

1. At rest (resting UPP)—with the patient and the urethra at rest
2. During stress (stress UPP)—by applying a defined provocation (e.g., cough, valsalva)
3. While voiding—this technique is fraught with technical difficulties, is rarely used in clinical practice, and will not be discussed any further

- The test is performed with the patient supine
- The zero pressure reference point taken as the superior edge of the symphysis pubis

- Correct placement and calibration can be ensured by asking the patient to contract the external sphincter
- Simultaneous recording of both urethral and intravesical pressures is essential to enable calculation of the urethral closure pressure
- Three profilometry techniques are in common use, and with each attention to detail is paramount

1. Brown-Wickham perfusion technique: works by measuring the pressure required to perfuse a catheter at a constant rate. A size 4–10 F, dual lumen (one for pressure measurement and the other for perfusion) catheter is inserted into the bladder. The catheter is perfused at a fixed rate (2–10 mL/min) and withdrawn very slowly to map the whole urethral pressure.

2. Balloon catheter technique: the pressure is detected by a small soft balloon mounted at the end of the catheter. More accurate but can be uncomfortable for the patient.

3. Catheter-mounted transducers: uses catheter tip transducer, but orientation of catheter can result in artifacts.

Although it is easier to perform UPP with the patient supine, this does not represent physiological conditions. Most patients complain of incontinence in the upright position or on standing. The measured UPP will be lower with the patient supine and should increase significantly (by about 20%) to aid continence in the upright position. Failure of such a rise may be seen in genuine stress incontinence due to intrinsic sphincter deficiency.

Stress UPP can only be performed with catheter-mounted transducers and is of limited value due to its decreased specificity. If required, it is best done with the patient in the upright position with a full bladder in an attempt to facilitate leakage. Following stress, the closure pressure decreases to less than $0 \, cmH_2O$ in the presence of genuine stress incontinence.

A number of variables can affect UPP and limit its reliability by abnormally elevating urethral pressures, including—

- Voluntary contractions of the external sphincter
- Contractions of the pelvic floor in the non-relaxed patient
- Urethral sensitivity
- Pain from transducer catheters or the balloon

Interpretation

Normal values
- Normal values for MUP in women are between 80 and 120 cmH$_2$O
- Younger women (<25 years of age) have a mean MUCP of 90 cmH$_2$O and this value decreases with age
- Postmenopausal women have a mean MUCP of 65 cmH$_2$O
- In men, MUP usually between 70 and 120 cmH$_2$O, and usually does not alter much with age
- The FPL may increase in the aging man due to increase in prostatic length, but tends to decrease in women
- Estrogens can increase FPL and MUP urethral length following menopause, but this improvement does not appear adequate to prevent stress leakage

Below is a normal female UPP, which is characterized by its symmetrical shape and the MUP is in the middle segment rather than at the level of the internal meatus (see Fig 5.4).

In males, however, there is a progressive increase in pressures throughout the length of the prostatic urethra, with the urethral pressure peaking in the membranous urethra, at the level of the external sphincter. The functional length in males is longer (6–7 cm) compared to females (3–4 cm).

Abnormalities of UPP
1. *Stress incontinence*
   - Typically there is a low urethral closure pressure which decreases further with bladder filling, along with an MUCP of <40 cmH$_2$O
   - FPL may decrease by up to 2 cm
   - Absence of a rise in urethral pressure upon assuming an upright position can often be noted
   - Demonstrable urine leakage on increasing intra-abdominal pressure, without any significant corresponding increase in urethral pressures
   - Initially, a low MUCP (<30 cmH$_2$O) was regarded as a predictor of poor outcome following retropubic suspension surgery (e.g., Burch colposuspension) and a sling procedure would be advocated

2. *Detrusor overactivity*
   - MUCP may be normal or even higher than expected

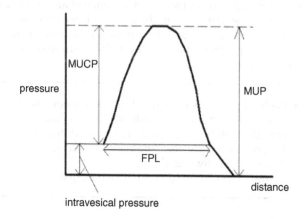

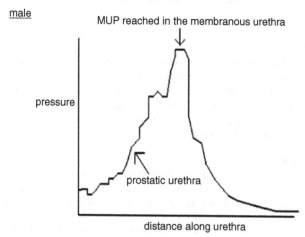

FIGURE 5.4. UPP of female (top) and male (below) urethra

- There tends to be a normal response to stress and adopting an upright position

3. *Urethral stenosis*
   - MUCP of >70 cmH₂O can be commonly found

4. *Detrusor–sphincter dyssynergia*
   - Instead of a drop in urethral pressures during voiding, there is an abnormal simultaneous increase

5. *Post-prostatectomy stress incontinence*
   - Associated features include an absence of any positive pressure in the prostatic urethra, normal pressure within the external sphincter, and a decrease in the functional length of the sphincteric segment (the main determinant of urinary incontinence)

- Useful in the assessment of urinary incontinence in conjunction with other urodynamic technique
- Fraught with technical and artifactual difficulties
- Absence of defined measurable parameters, but trends may be clinically useful
- Routine use restricted to a few departments

(f) VIDEOURODYNAMICS

Overview
Videourodynamics (VUDS) combines standard cystometry combined with synchronous imaging of the lower urinary tract. In the majority of cases simple cystometry is sufficient to investigate most patients with LUTS, but the advantage of VUDS is in its enabling the clinician to simultaneously study the anatomy and physiology of voiding dysfunction.

Indications
In the main, the indications for VUDS are much the same as those for standard cystometry. On occasions, additional anatomical information may be valuable, and potential indications include—

- Investigation of stress incontinence in women, especially following failed surgical intervention
- To define the level of suspected bladder outlet obstruction in younger men (prostatic obstruction is uncommon in the younger male)
- Assessment of the neuropathic bladder, especially if detrusor–sphincter dyssynergia and/or ureteric reflux is suspected
- Investigation of post-prostatectomy stress incontinence
- Children in whom invasive therapy for voiding dysfunction is being considered

Technique
This technique is similar to conventional cystometry, but with the addition of a radioopaque filling medium, video recorder, and

X-ray equipment. Some authors have used real-time ultrasound scanning, arguing its distinct advantage in abolishing the radiation risk and providing adequate bladder images. However, the other anatomical information obtained by USS is limited and it has not gained widespread acceptance.

- Most units use 200–250 mL of water-soluble contrast, and complete bladder filling using saline
- During voiding, females will often have to void standing up to allow fluoroscopic imaging of the lower urinary tract

Interpretation

Normal voiding
Principles of pressure and pressure-flow analysis are identical to conventional cystometry. However additional findings may be recorded:

- Bladder—initial residual volume, shape and position, trabeculation, diverticula, ureteric reflux, fistula, and post-void residual
- Bladder neck—shape, descent of during stress or voiding
- Urethra—"milking back" on voluntary inhibition of voiding, stenosis, diverticula
- Demonstration of leakage

During filling, the bladder neck and urethra should remain closed. In some older women, the bladder neck may open on coughing or valsalva. On voiding, the bladder base may exhibit minimal descent, the bladder neck opens widely and normal voiding occurs through a relaxed and patent urethra. The bladder should empty to completion.

Stopping the urine flow voluntarily, results in contractions of the pelvic floor which "milk back" the urine into the bladder and the bladder neck closes.

Common abnormalities on VUDS
1. *Incompetent bladder neck*
    - Bladder neck opening during filling or on coughing is abnormal in men and younger women. This may be due to involuntary detrusor contractions or bladder neck incompetence

2. *Failure of bladder neck opening*
    - May be due to bladder neck stenosis, detrusor–sphincter dyssynergia, or a hypotonic bladder

- In the hypotonic bladder, pressure studies will confirm a low Pdet during voiding
- Higher voiding bladder pressures are noted with bladder neck stenosis and detrusor–sphincter dyssynergia

3. *Stress incontinence*
   - Stress leakage may occur secondary to either urethral/bladder neck hypermobility or intrinsic sphincter deficiency, or a combination of both
   - Descent of the bladder neck is easily demonstrated on VUDS and can be graded (see below)
   - In patients with significant intrinsic sphincter deficiency, there is minimal bladder neck descent on straining and prolonged leakage through an open urethra is the typical finding
   - Blaivas and Olsson have proposed a classification system for genuine stress incontinence (GSI) based on the VUDS conclusions

   Type 0—history of GSI but no leakage demonstrated on VUDS (possibly due to voluntary sphincteric contractions)
   Type I—at rest the closed bladder neck is situated at or above the inferior margin of the symphysis pubis. On coughing there is demonstrable leakage. The bladder neck and proximal urethra open, but bladder neck descent is <2 cm
   Type IIA—as above, except descent on coughing is >2 cm and there is an obvious cystourethrocoele
   Type IIB—bladder neck closed at rest but lies below inferior margin of symphysis pubis. On coughing, leakage occurs with or without bladder neck descent
   Type III—abnormally open bladder neck and proximal urethra during bladder filling

4. *Ureteric reflux*
   - Seen during voiding
   - May be unilateral or bilateral
   - Often associated with a neurogenic bladder

Limitations
- Radiation exposure to patient and staff
- Cost of equipment and extra technical support (e.g., radiographer)
- Additional fluoroscopic information may add little to cystometric data
- Lack of privacy and women having to void standing up

- Most comprehensive method of assessment of voiding dysfunction
- Excellent anatomical and physiological information
- Gold standard for the evaluation of stress incontinence

(g) AMBULATORY URODYNAMICS

Overview
Conventional urodynamics (UDS) has its disadvantages. It is—

- Non-physiological
- Prone to artifacts due to a number of factors
- Requires a laboratory setting of the test with the patient having to void on demand
- Based on rapid bladder filling by an indwelling catheter
- Can overestimate decreased bladder compliance and underdiagnose detrusor overactivity in up to 50% of cases

Ambulatory urodynamics (AUDS) has become an established method of investigating lower urinary tract function in a more physiological manner, by enabling natural bladder filling and allowing the patient to undertake their normal activities to provoke troublesome urinary symptoms.

Indications
- Investigation of incontinence or troublesome LUTS where conventional UDS has been normal
- Situations where conventional UDS may be unsuitable
- Assessment of the neuropathic bladder where a slow physiological bladder filling is required
- In research studies testing the efficacy of therapies for LUTS

Technique
- The study requires 3–4 hours
- The patient is fitted with bladder pressure transducer catheters within the bladder and rectum which are secured and calibrated
- These remain connected to a battery-operated portable storage device throughout the duration of the study
- Patients are allowed to move around the hospital till at least three voiding cycles have been completed

- Some centers ask patients to perform progressively strenuous activities in an attempt to simulate daily activities and elicit incontinence (e.g., sitting, walking, running, or exercise)
- Patients can void into a uroflowmeter
- The use of a patient diary considerably improves the detailed analysis of events occurring during AUDS and is strongly recommended
- On completion of the test, the data on the portable recording device can be analyzed

Typical events occurring during the filling phase are detrusor contractions, urethral relaxations, and episodes of urgency and incontinence. Patient participation is essential for complete analysis of AUDS, as they need to record the following using either an event marker button or a frequency voiding chart:

- Time and number of voluntary voids
- Episodes of urgency
- Episodes of discomfort or pain
- Provocative maneuvers
- Time and volume of fluid intake
- Time and volume of urinary leakage
- Time and number of pad changes

Interpretation
The principles of analysis of the traces is similar to those used in conventional cystometry. However, certain notable differences have been noted between measurements obtained from conventional and ambulatory UDS.

1. *Detrusor overactivity* (see Fig 5.5)

  - AUDS is significantly more sensitive in the detection of involuntary detrusor contraction during the filling phase compared to conventional UDS
  - The more prolonged and physiological nature of AUDS may well account for this seeming superiority. While this would appear to strengthen the case for ambulatory studies, it is noteworthy that this difference is seen in both symptomatic and asymptomatic patients. Between 30% and 69% of asymptomatic patients were noted to have evidence of detrusor overactivity on AUDS analysis. It may be that phasic detrusor contractions is a "normal" finding and of no clinical significance in the absence of symptoms

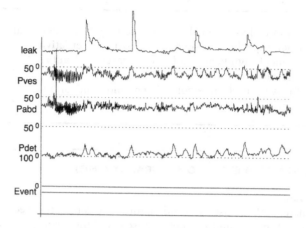

FIGURE 5.5. Ambulatory UDS trace showing episodic urine leakage associated with increases in detrusor pressure (detrusor overactivity) (with permission from *Urodynamics*, Abrams, Springer, 1997, 97)

2. *Bladder compliance*
   - Patients shown to have low compliance (therefore high end-fill pressure) on conventional UDS, often have lower pressures (and better compliance) on AUDS
   - In fact, the loss of compliance seen in the former is probably replaced by phasic detrusor contractions seen in the latter study
   - It is likely that the rapid bladder filling during conventional studies is responsible, in part at least, for the loss of compliance

3. *Bladder outflow obstruction*
   - Similarly, rapid bladder filling (and possible overstretching) during conventional cystometry may alter the contractile properties of the detrusor, resulting in decreased voiding pressures
   - Male and female patients undergoing AUDS show higher voiding pressures, improved flow rates, and decreased voided volumes compared to conventional studies

AUDS also demonstrates an increased ability to diagnose a functional abnormality (detrusor overactivity or urethral sphincter deficiency) associated with urinary incontinence.

- A more physiological means of testing the lower urinary tract, especially in suspected detrusor overactivity
- Clinical significance of the apparent advantages are unclear
- Invasive and time-consuming and clinical utility is restricted

---

(h) SPHINCTER ELECTROMYOGRAPHY (EMG)

Overview

Sphincter EMG is used in urodynamics to evaluate the electrical activity of the striated sphincter muscle and the pelvic floor striated muscles that aid urinary continence. The functional unit in EMG is the motor unit, which comprises a single motor neurone and the muscle fiber it innervates. At rest, the contracted external urethral sphincteric (EUS) gives rise to low amplitude electrical activity on the EMG. EMG alone gives useful information about EUS function, but it is most valuable when done in conjunction with cystometry to particularly determine the functional coordination between bladder and sphincter activity.

Indications

The precise role of EMG has not been clearly defined in current urodynamic practice, and it has been argued that it provides little information beyond what has been obtained following a thorough clinical neurological examination of the perineum and lower limbs, and videourodynamics. It may, however, be a useful diagnostic test for the evaluation of a patient with voiding dysfunction if a neuropathic cause for the patient's disorder is not immediately apparent. The following clinical situations may be suitable for EMG studies:

- Neuropathic patients with suspected detrusor–sphincter dyssynergia (e.g., spinal cord injury, Parkinson's disease, multiple sclerosis, or motor neuron disease)
- Assessment of voiding dysfunction following radical pelvic or spinal surgery
- Young women with voiding difficulties or recurrent episodes of retention (e.g., urethral stenosis/Fowler's syndrome)
- Children with dysfunctional voiding—can also be used to provide biofeedback during pelvic floor relaxation training

Technique
- EMG usually undertaken in combination with other urodynamic techniques
- Can be performed with the patient supine, sitting, or standing
- Electrical activity can be picked up either by needle or surface electrodes
- In the female, the needle electrodes are placed directly in the EUS, located about 1 inch in from the external meatus. Needles placed at the 1 o'clock and 11 o'clock position provide the most reliable information
- In males, the EUS is reached by inserting the electrodes between the base of the scrotum and the rectum, parallel to the rectum, about 2 inches deep to skin
- If placement is correct, the EMG should demonstrate increased muscle activity with voluntary tightening of the EUS and decreased muscle activity upon relaxation
- Surface electrodes, including skin patch and anal plug electrodes, are applied to the skin surface close to the sphincter and therefore detect electrical activity from groups of adjacent motor units. Patches are placed on either side of the external anal sphincter, as close to the rectal mucosa as possible, at the 3 and 9 o'clock position. Surface electrodes are less uncomfortable but have decreased reliability and reproducibility compared to their needle counterparts
- Electrical activity is either displayed graphically on a monitor screen or audibly on special speakers and studies interpreted in real time, as they are being performed

Standard kinesiological EMG does not diagnose neuropathy but simply demonstrates the effects of neuropathy on the EUS. However, motor unit EMG is another type of sophisticated neurophysiological investigation which can accurately detect denervation or myopathy in the striated pelvic floor musculature. This is more invasive and requires an experienced neurologist with considerable experience in such techniques.

Interpretation
The International Continence Society has not specified normal findings for sphincter EMG. However if EMG and cystometry are performed together, under normal circumstances—

- There is constant electrical activity within the EUS and pelvic floor at rest, which increases progressively with bladder filling (guarding reflex)

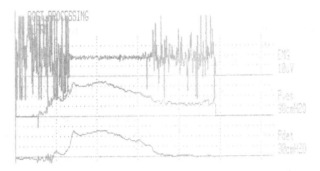

FIGURE 5.6. Simultaneous EMG and cystometry showing a normal response—increased electrical EMG activity during the filling phase followed by electrical silence during voiding (Courtesy of Mr C Betts, Hope Hospital, Salford)

- EMG activity peaks just before voiding
- During filling, the EMG activity may be increased due to voluntary squeezing of the urethra, straining, or involuntary abnormal detrusor contractions
- The EMG becomes silent immediately prior to voiding, representing relaxation of the EUS and pelvic musculature (Fig. 5.6)

Any EUS activity during micturition is abnormal unless the patient is voluntarily trying to stop urine flow. EMG activity returns when the bladder is empty. An abnormal EMG from either the failure of the sphincter to relax or from increased muscle activity during voiding may be due to detrusor–sphincter dyssynergia, seen in patients with a true neuropathic bladder due to multiple sclerosis, spinal cord injury, and other neurological lesions. Additionally in the absence of an obvious neurological pathology, increased abnormal spontaneous EMG activity during voiding may be seen in patients with pelvic floor hyperactivity (e.g., Fowler's syndrome) resulting in urine retention in young women. EMG results must always be correlated with patient symptoms, physical examination, and other urodynamic findings.

Chapter 6
Other

(a) TRANSRECTAL ULTRASOUND OF THE PROSTATE

Overview
Transrectal ultrasound of the prostate (TRUS) is the single most commonly performed procedure on the prostate. Although traditionally used to direct prostate needle biopsies, it also provides useful information regarding prostate volume, anatomy and aids in treatment planning.

Indications

Prostate cancer
- Direct prostate biopsies for the detection of CAP
  - If PSA > 4 ng/mL (some authors suggest a lower cut-off of 2.5 ng/mL)
  - Abnormal DRE
  - Presence of high-grade prostatic intraepithelial neoplasia (PIN) in previous biopsies—between 27% and 79% will have evidence of CAP in repeat biopsies
  - Rising PSA or palpable abnormality following definitive treatment
- Local staging in established prostate cancer
- Treatment planning (for thermal coil placement or interstitial radioactive seed placement on brachytherapy)

Benign disease
- To measure prostate gland volume
- Assessment in chronic prostatitis
- Evaluation of male infertility (to exclude prostatic duct or seminal vesicle obstruction)

Technique

Patient preparation

TRUS can safely be performed as an office procedure. Some institutions advocate the routine use of a pre-procedure cleansing enema to decrease rectal content. TRUS is contraindicated in the presence of a UTI and patients on anticoagulants must be advised to stop therapy for 2–3 days. Given the high incidence of transient post-TRUS bacteraemia (up to 73%) and risk of sepsis, all patients must be given prophylactic antibiotics. Protocols may vary according to local policy, but a broad-spectrum antibiotic (e.g., three oral doses of a quinolone or a single dose of IV gentamicin) will usually suffice, but high-risk patients (e.g., valvular heart disease) must receive a penicillin-based antibiotic as well. The procedure can be performed with the patient in the lateral decubitus, lithotomy, or knee-chest position. A careful digital examination to assess anal tone, rectal contents, and prostatic morphology is mandatory.

Equipment

Most procedures are performed using a 6–7.5-MHz transrectal US transducer which can scan in the transverse as well as the longitudinal/sagittal plane. Transverse images better demonstrate prostatic symmetry and lateral capsular anatomy. The longitudinal is used for biopsies due to the easier visualisation of the prostate base and apex. A spring-loaded Tru-Cut type 18 G biopsy gun is used for prostate biopsy.

Anesthesia

Traditionally, six-core sextant biopsies were usually performed without anesthesia. More recently however, the discomfort associated with the general trends toward increased biopsy core numbers has resulted in greater use of local anesthesia. Various methods have been described, including—

- Peri-prostatic nerve blockade provides the best anesthesia (10 mL of 1% lidocaine)
- Intra-rectal 2% lidocaine jelly
- Entonox gas inhalation
- Oral anti-inflammatories

Interpretation

A real-time interpretation by an experienced physician provides greatest yield from a TRUS examination. A systematic approach is vital.

A **B**

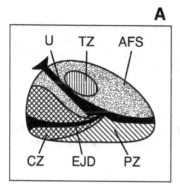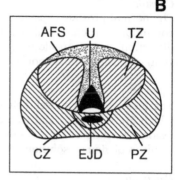

FIGURE 6.1. Zonal anatomy of the prostate gland—(**A**) sagittal and (**B**) transverse view (with permission from Campbell's *Urology*, Saunders, 2000, **3044–3045**) (TZ = transitional zone, CZ = central zone, PZ = peripheral zone, U = urethra, EJD = ejaculatory ducts, AFS = anterior fibromuscular stroma)

Prostate zones (see Fig 6.1)

BPH is limited to the transitional zone (TZ) of the prostate which lies anteriorly. The increasing size of the TZ usually appears hypoechoic and compresses the more posteriorly placed central (CZ) and peripheral zones (PZ). While it is relatively easy to distinguish the TZ from the PZ, the CZ is not easy identified on TRUSS.

Prostate cancer

TRUS detects 50% more patients with CAP than DRE in asymptomatic patients. The appearance of CAP on TRUS is a heterogenous phenomenon. Cancers usually arise within the PZ, but up to 20% can be located in the TZ. The classic hypoechoic area in the PZ is not always seen and many cancers are isoechoic and only detectable from systematic biopsies. Suspicious palpable nodules on rectal examination are more likely to appear as hypoechoic lesions. Generally, up to 70% of tumors are hypoechoic, while the rest are indistinguishable from surrounding prostatic tissue (isoechoic). TZ cancers are more likely to be isoechoic. There appears to be no relationship between the tumor echogenicity and the subsequent Gleason score. Prostatic inflammation, infarcts, atrophy, and hypertrophy can also result in the appearance of hypoechoic lesions.

Capsule
The normal prostate capsule is a symmetrical and well-defined, continuous structure which appears hyperechoic. Breaches or distortion of the capsule (e.g., secondary to local tumor extension) can usually be demonstrated on TRUSS.

Cysts
These can be seen as well-defined, smooth, spherical structures which are echo-poor and cast an acoustic shadow beyond the lesion. Puncture of these lesions with the biopsy gun will often result in obvious resolution.

Calcification
Calcification is frequently seen in the interface between the TZ and PZ and usually is a feature of BPH. Calcification can also be associated with prostatitis and prostatic malignancies, although this is generally regarded as a non-specific finding.

Seminal vesicles and ejaculatory ducts
The seminal vesicles (SV) can easily be seen on the posterior surface of the bladder, just superior to the prostate. Although usually symmetrical in appearance, asymmetry is a common non-diagnostic finding. Other causes of asymmetry or SV dilatation include ejaculatory duct obstruction and invasion by CAP. An A–P diameter >15 mm and a length >35 mm is typical of SV obstruction. The SV may be absent or atrophic in patients with congenital absence of the vas. TRUS-aided SV aspiration can help detect increased sperm concentration in the SV, which is suggestive of an obstructive pathology.

Prostate biopsy
Prostate biopsy remains a controversial issue with no standardized consensus with regard to technique, number of biopsy cores and region of prostate to be biopsied.

The larger the gland, the lesser the likelihood of CAP detection and the greater the false-negative rate. The rate of CAP detection increases from 23% to 31% in glands >50 cc to 38–50% in glands measuring <30 cc. Generally, more biopsy cores must be taken in prostates which are larger on TRUS volume estimation.

In patients undergoing TRUS biopsy for the first time, TZ-directed biopsies are not recommended due to the poor detection rate. However, during subsequent biopsies, a conscious attempt must be made to obtain tissue from the midline, peri-urethral regions. The TZ is best sampled by transurethral resection.

Directed biopsies: biopsies directed toward a palpable nodule or from an abnormal-looking area on TRUS generally results in a poorer yield (cancer detection rate of just over 50%) due to the varied appearance of prostate cancer on TRUS.

Sextant technique: the sextant biopsy technique has been the traditional gold standard method till recent years, with a sensitivity rate of approximately 70%. Three core biopsies are taken from both lobes of the prostate in the midlobe parasagittal plane at the base, middle, and apex. Some authors have argued that the biopsies must be directed more laterally to increase diagnostic yield, since over 80% of cancers are located in the posterolateral aspect of the PZ of the prostate gland. The estimated sensitivity of laterally directed sextant biopsies is between 75% and 85%. The sextant technique is notoriously inadequate for the detection of TZ cancers, with a sensitivity of around 30%.

Five region biopsies: this protocol with 13–18 cores increased the detection rate by 35% when compared to standard, mid-lobar sextant biopsies. Although there is little doubt that increasing the number of cores is likely to result in a superior cancer detection rate, it does not seem to decrease the requirement for repeat biopsies. In a five-region technique, in addition to the standard sextant regions, further cores are taken from the far lateral and midline regions of the gland.

A number of other modifications have been described, primarily with the effect of increasing the number of cores and directing them more laterally, with a resultant improvement in sensitivities of between 20% and 38% compared to sextant biopsies.

Saturation biopsies: usually performed under a general anesthetic and result in the taking of 20–30 core biopsies.

Repeat biopsies: If the first set of biopsies is negative, repeated biopsies can be recommended if concern persists regarding the presence of a malignancy (e.g., rising PSA, abnormal DRE, presence of high-grade PIN). The second biopsy should ideally include a biopsy technique adopted for the initial procedure plus additional TZ and lateral region biopsies. A detection rate of about 10–38% has been reported in cases with a negative first set of biopsies. If initial biopsies confirm the existence of high-grade PIN, immediate re-biopsy is indicated since as many as 27–79% of prostates harbor a concomitant cancer. Not infrequently a patient may undergo a third set of prostate biopsies with quoted CAP detection rates of between 5% and 30%.

Drawbacks
1. Invasive and uncomfortable
2. Complications
   - Hematuria, rectal bleeding, or hematospermia (>50%)
   - UTI/ sepsis (2%)
   - Urinary retention (1–2%)
3. Inaccuracies in cancer staging (sensitivity for detection of extra-capsular penetration is around 60%)
4. Imaging prone to artifacts (e.g., secondary to air, calcification, rapid movement)
5. Vasovagal episodes due to vagal nerve stimulation (<5%)

(b) URINARY STONE ANALYSIS

Overview
Stone disease is common and up to 50% of patients with at least one stone will experience further recurrences. It is now accepted that evidence-based medical intervention is the only approach likely to make a significant impact on the incidence, and more importantly, the recurrence rates of this disease. Intervention requires reliable stone composition information combined with relevant blood and urine analyses. While other parameters, including urine pH, urinary crystals, and radiological appearance may suggest a certain stone type, appropriate stone analysis is the most accurate method to determine stone composition. Stone analysis complements, but does not replace, blood and urine analysis in overall metabolic assessment of the stone former and all patients should have at least one stone analyzed.

A variety of crystalline components can be identified accurately. In whole stones, separate analysis of the nucleus from the rest of the stone will often show a difference in chemical composition. Traditionally, chemical stone analysis has been poorly performed in many laboratories, resulting in misguided diagnosis and inappropriate therapy. Advances in recent techniques have improved diagnostic accuracy.

Indications

All patients should undergo at least one stone analysis to enable documentation of baseline stone composition. The arguments supporting routine analysis are—

- Identification of chemical constituents help define risk factors
- Finding of a stone constituent points to a specific diagnosis (e.g., cystine)
- May indicate a change in urinary environment (e.g., as a result of surgery)
- To help identify regional trends in stone disease
- To distinguish between genuine stones and artifacts which may be submitted for analysis (e.g., inorganic materials, metallic objects, polystyrene)

A repeat stone analysis is indicated—

- If there is a change in urine composition
- Following prophylaxis or medical treatment
- Following a change in dietary habits, environment, or diseases, which can all be expected to have influenced the stone composition

Techniques

Stone analysis must be performed soon after passage or removal of stone and interpreted in the light of any changes to therapy. A brief summary of available techniques is given in the table below (Table 6.1).

Interpretation

The standard frequencies of urinary stones are listed below (Table 6.2).

- Stone analysis provides a diagnosis, identifies risk factors, and directs treatment
- All patients must undergo at least one stone analysis
- Calcium-containing stones most common (>80%)
- Infrared spectroscopy with wet chemical analysis is standard regime
- Substandard analysis is misleading

TABLE 6.1. Stone analysis techniques

Method	Comment
Wet chemical analysis	Most widely used technique in routine hospital laboratories
	Commercial kits available
	Suitably prepared stone solution undergoes routine chemical analysis (similar to blood and urine)
	Qualitative and semi-quantitative
	Relatively poor performance
	False positives and false negatives common
	Requires 10–15 mg of stone material
	Accuracy worse for mixed (compared to single component) stones
	Often unable to detect rarer constituents
X-ray diffraction	Identification of the unique diffraction patterns produced following bombardment of stone powder by monochromatic X-rays
	Greater accuracy than wet chemical analysis
	Expensive
	Time-consuming
	Minor and non-crystalline components may be missed in up to 20% of cases
Infrared spectroscopy	Fast becoming the gold standard technique
	Stone powder is exposed to infrared radiation
	Rapid
	Relatively inexpensive
	Will detect rare, artifactual and non-crystalline components
	Can be performed on small amount of material (>0.1 mg)
Scanning electron microscopy with energy dispersion	Non-destructive technique
	Components can be visualised without alteration
	Phosphate component may be missed
	Not widely available
Thermogravimetry	Detects pattern of weight change when stone material is heated to 1,000°C
	Requires specialized equipment
	Large amounts of stone matter needed
	Some compounds (e.g., purines, silica) may be missed
Polarizing microscopy	Microscopy of segments of a stone to reveal internal structure
	Unable to identify small amounts of crystalline matter
	Operator dependent

TABLE 6.2. Frequency of urinary stones

Stone Composition	Frequency (%)	Comment
Calcium	80	Calcium-containing stones are
Oxalate	35	most common; further
Phosphate	10	metabolic testing may reveal
Oxalate + phosphate	35	hypercalciuria, hyperoxaluria, hypocitraturia, or hyperuricosuria
Struvite	10	Infection stones—frequently present as staghorn stones in alkaline urine
Uric acid	8	Associated with an acidic urine (pH < 5.5) and occurs in men with a high purine intake, gout, myeloproliferative disorder, or weight loss
Cystine	1	Diagnostic of cystinuria—an autosomal recessive inborn error of metabolism
Others (xanthine, non-crystalline, etc.)	1	Xanthine stones—congenital deficiency of xanthine oxidase or allopurinol intake Indinavir stones—seen in patients on protease inhibitors (for treatment of HIV infection) Silica—in patients on long-term silica-containing antacids

(c) PAD TEST FOR URINARY INCONTINENCE

Overview

Stress leakage is—

- Subjective
- Not always readily demonstrated on UDS
- Degree of urine loss may not be reliably quantified by UDS

Pad testing is a reasonably reliable, non-invasive method of detecting and quantifying urine loss under standard and reproducible conditions.

Indications
- Detect stress leakage if UDS normal
- Quantify degree of urinary leakage
- Measure treatment outcome

Technique
The test must not be performed if the patient is menstruating or has concurrent UTI. Many variations on a central theme have been described.

- A FVC must be completed prior to the study
- Test duration must be a minimum of 1 hour for hospital tests (or 24–48 hours for home tests)
- A bladder volume of two-thirds normal capacity is ideal. The bladder may be allowed to fill normally or can be filled using a catheter
- The patient must not void during the 1-hour test
- The test commences upon application of a pre-weighed dry pad (inside waterproof underpants)
- Some centers advocate further bladder filling to stress the system by asking the patients to drink 500 mL of water during the first 15 min
- If physically able, the patient is then asked to perform a series of activities to simulate common daily tasks, which must include—
  - Sitting (for up to 30 min)
  - Standing up from sitting (>10 times)
  - Bending (>5 times)
  - Coughing (>10 times)
  - Climbing stairs (at least one flight)
  - Running on the spot (for >1 min)
  - Hand-washing (for >1 min)
- If patient unable to inhibit voiding, the test may be repeated
- The test duration may be extended by 1-hour slots, but in practice patients are often unable to hold off micturition if the test period is prolonged
- Patients on home pad testing (24–48 h) are instructed to collect all pads in an airtight container
- The pad(s) are weighed after completion of the test period

In certain situations, oral pyridium can be used to stain the urine orange, which will help distinguish urine leakage from vaginal discharge.

Interpretation
The normal limit of pad weight gain is—

* <1.4 g per hour
* <8 g per 24 h (for home testing)

Values greater than these are presumed to be secondary to urine leakage.

A negative 1-hour test may need to be repeated, especially if the patient continues to complain of stress leakage. The prolonged 24–48-hour test is inherently more accurate and reproducible compared than the hour-long test.

(d) LAPAROSCOPY FOR UNDESCENDED TESTIS

Overview
Cryptorchidism or undescended testis (UDT)—

* Has an incidence of 3–5% (at birth) and 0.8% (age of 1 year)
* May affect one or both (20% bilateral) testes
* Requires mandatory evaluation due to concerns about malignant change and decreased fertility in the cryptorchid testis

Laparoscopy is a safe and well-established therapeutic technique in modern day adult and pediatric urology. However, it is also a diagnostic tool and its most extensive application has been in the management of the impalpable cryptorchid testis with an accuracy for testicular localisation approaching 100%.

Indications
* Establish the presence and location of impalpable testis
* Remove an intra-abdominal testis (laparoscopic orchidectomy) not deemed suitable for orchidopexy, whose presence and location is already known (e.g., following US or MRI scan)

Technique and findings
* The ideal time for surgery is between 12 and 18 months of age (although laparoscopy is safe in infants as young as 3 months)
* Performed as a day-case procedure if uncomplicated
* Informed consent is obtained from the patient's guardian
* Performed under a general anesthetic, with the patient supine

- Following Veress needle puncture or open access (e.g., Hasson technique), the peritoneal cavity is insufflated to a pressure of around 10 mmHg
- A single 2- or 5- mm port is placed through the umbilicus
- Careful inspection of the abdomen and pelvis is made using a 2–5-mm laparoscope
- Additional ports may be required depending on the subsequent procedure

One of four clinical scenarios may be encountered (Table 6.3).

- Complications are uncommon (<1%)
  - Intra-abdominal organ injury
  - Bleeding
  - Infection
  - Respiratory complications
  - Trauma to vas and cord structures

- Accurate in detection of impalpable testis
- Dual-purpose, minimally invasive procedure (diagnosis and therapeutic)
- Avoids laparotomy and therefore decreases morbidity
- Any other imaging technique to locate the testis would require a general anesthetic as well

---

TABLE 6.3. Possible outcomes during pediatric laparoscopy for UDT

Laparoscopic Finding	Comments and Action
Blind ending vas and spermatic vessels above the internal inguinal ring (44%)	Vanishing testis (possibly due to ischemia in fetal life) → no further action is required
Intra-abdominal testis located either adjacent to the internal inguinal ring, in the retroperitoneum or the pelvis (36%)	If atrophic → consider laparoscopic orchidectomy Assess viability for orchidopexy— either open or laparoscopic; one- or two-stage procedure
Vas and spermatic cord seen entering the internal inguinal ring (20%)	Testis likely to be in the inguinal canal → open exploration of inguinal canal
Inability to visualize either the testis or the spermatic vessels laparoscopically (<1%)	→ open exploration mandatory

(e) ASPIRATION OF RENAL CYST

Overview
Renal cysts are common (70% of all asymptomatic) and usually of little clinical significance. Given the improved accuracy of US and CT imaging in the evaluation and categorization of renal masses, renal cyst aspirations have now become a relatively uncommon occurrence.

Indications
Although there are no absolute indications for renal cyst puncture (RCP), a variety of relative indications exist, including—

- Evaluation of an indeterminate renal mass (if US and CT inconclusive)
- Relief of local symptoms (e.g., loin pain) attributed to the cyst
- Abnormal calcification within cyst wall
- Unexplained fever or hematuria with apparent cyst

Technique
Contraindications and patient preparation are identical to those described for nephrostomy insertion (see Chapter 3g—Nephrostogram). A single dose of a prophylactic antibiotic agent must be administered.

- A 21–22-gauge needle is inserted percutaneously under local anesthesia (1% lidocaine)
- Laparoscopic cyst de-roofing requires a general anesthetic
- When using a needle, cyst localization is achieved using a combination of USS (most common), CT, or fluoroscopy
- Once the cyst is punctured, the fluid is aspirated
  - Simple cyst fluid is clear and straw-colored
  - Blood-stained aspirate may be due to—
    (i)   Hemorrhage into a simple cyst
    (ii) Traumatic puncture
    (iii) Hematoma
    (iv) Complex/malignant cyst
- Although many operators will terminate the procedure at this stage, injection of 1–2 ml of contrast into the cyst may help clarify the anatomy
- If no aspiration is possible, in spite of correct placement, the mass is assumed to be solid in consistency (about 25% will eventually prove to be malignant)

Supplementary techniques

1. *Renal cyst aspiration and sclerosing*: once needle access into the cyst is achieved, a guidewire is advanced, the needle replaced with a pig-tail catheter, and the cyst aspirated to dryness. To reduce the high risk of recurrence, injecting the cyst with a cytotoxic sclerosing agent is advisable. Such agents include pure alcohol, sotradecol, or tetracycline (100mg). The volume of the sclerosing agent injected is no more than half of the volume of aspirate. Care must be taken to avoid extravasation of sclerosant into the retroperitoneum, collecting system, or vascular compartment. The sclerosant is drained away completely after 15 minutes.

2. *Renal cyst aspiration and examination of contents*: the cyst contents are aspirated and examined for—
- Biochemical content: protein, electrolytes, fat
- Micro-organisms
- Abnormal cytology

3. *Laparoscopic de-roofing of cysts*: large solitary cysts, and occasionally multiple cysts (e.g., polycystic kidneys) can be treated using the laparoscopic approach. The cyst wall is completely excised and the base and edges can be fulgurated using diathermy or argon beam coagulator. Any abnormal-looking areas can be biopsied for clarification. This technique does not adversely affect global renal function.

Limitations
- Invasive procedure
- Risk of abscess formation
- Perirenal hematoma
- Sclerosing agents can cause discomfort
- Theoretical risk of causing tumor seeding
- Does not prevent new cyst formation

(f) URETHRAL SWABS

Overview

Urethral swabs are taken primarily for the diagnosis of sexually transmitted infections (STI) in men. Typical symptoms include any of the following:

- Urethral discharge
- Urethral pain

- Dysuria
- Non-specific symptoms suggestive of pelvic inflammatory disease

Microbiological analysis using urethral swabs is easy, safe, and is reasonably sensitive in males. In females however examining a gram-stained smear from an isolated urethral swab sample is often insufficient to make the diagnosis, and a full pelvic bacteriological screen including a high vaginal and cervical specimen is recommended.

- The most common pathogens are *Neisseria gonorrhea, Chlamydia trachomatis*, and *Trichomonas vaginalis*
- Furthermore, these organisms often coexist in synergy (e.g., 20% of males and 40% of females with *gonorrhea* also have a concurrent *Chlamydia* infection)
- Positive results should prompt treatment of patient and their sexual partners

Indications
- Urethral discharge
- Urethral pain and dysuria
- Chronic lower UTI refractory to antibiotics
- Symptoms of pelvic inflammatory disease in women
- Symptoms suggestive of chronic lower urinary tract symptoms (e.g., chronic epididymo-orchitis or prostatitis)

Technique
Specimen collection prior to commencement of antimicrobial therapy provides the greatest yield. No specific contraindications exist as such:

- A cotton, rayon, or dacron-tipped, wire-mounted swab is ideal. In females, a non-bristled cytology brush may be used. A separate swab is used for each different pathogen being tested for. In addition, if testing for *T. vaginalis*, two swabs are required (see below)
- A first early-morning sample, prior to micturition, is ideal but often impractical
- Any exudate can be expressed by "milking" the urethra
- If material is not readily obtained, the swab is inserted 3–4 cm in to the anterior urethra
- Leave the swab in for a few seconds to allow saturation with the exudate (*N. gonorrhea* inhabits the exudate)

- If testing for *Chlamydia*, the swab must be rotated through 360° a few times to dislodge epithelial cells (*Chlamydia* is strictly intracellular within the urethral epithelial cells)
- Swabs for *N. gonorrhea* are transported in a container neutral agar, while *Chlamydia* containers have a special sucrose–phosphate medium with 5% fetal calf serum (often with added gentamicin to inhibit other microorganisms). One of the two swabs taken for *T. vaginalis* identification is placed in a tube containing 0.5 ml of sterile normal saline and transported immediately for direct wet mounts and cultures
- Swabs must be kept at room temperature and refrigeration should be avoided due to the susceptibility of these organisms to fluctuations in temperature
- Specimen must be sent to the laboratory within 6 hours, as the recovery rate of microorganisms decreases after this period
- The traditional method of diagnosis is to examine a gram-stained preparation of the urethral swab smear for identification of the pathogen. Newer techniques have improved detection rates

---

- Efficient method of diagnosing STI
- High sensitivity (79–97%) and specificity (87–99%)
- A negative test does not necessarily exclude infection, especially with persistent symptoms
- Recent urine based tests for *Chlamydia* and *T. vaginalis* have superseded urethral sampling

---

(g) BLADDER CATHETERIZATION

Overview

Bladder catheterization ranks as one of the most frequently performed manipulative procedures in the urinary tract. While it primarily remains a therapeutic technique for patients in urinary retention, a number of diagnostic applications exist as well:

- Measurement of residual urine volume
- Collection of reliable urine sample for analysis
- Estimation of urine output
- Radiographic procedures (e.g., cystography, MCUG)
- Urodynamic purposes (e.g., filling and pressure-measuring catheter)

Types of catheters
The choice of catheter depends on the precise purpose, since there is so much variability in catheter size, type of material, tip shape, and number of lumens see table 6.4.

- Short-term catheters can remain indwelling for up to 4 weeks
- Long-term catheters should be replaced every 12 weeks

Size
Measured according to the Charriere French (F) gauge, where 1F = 0.33 outer diameter.

- A size 12F catheter will have an outer diameter of 4 mm
- For most standard purposes a size 14–18F is adequate
- Size of 20–24F is used for bladder irrigation or washout (for debris, mucus, or clots)
- Male length catheters are longer (40–45 cm) compared to those used in females (20–26 cm)

Tip shape
- A straight, floppy-tip standard catheter is suitable for most cases
- The upward-deflected stiff Coude tip is better for negotiating the high bladder neck or the occlusive prostatic urethra
- The whistle-tip catheter, with an end opening, is often better suited for the washout of larger bladder clots

Lumen
Catheters may be—

- Single lumen (e.g., intermittent self-catheterization, urodynamics)
- Double lumen (e.g., most standard catheters)
- Triple lumen (e.g., irrigating catheters)

Triple-lumen catheters have smaller outflow lumens than the corresponding-size double-lumen catheters.

   Complications of bladder catheterization include—

- Infections
- Urethra—discharge, trauma, stricture, catheter hypospadias
- Discomfort

TABLE 6.4. Catheters

Type	Nature	Uses	Comments
Plastic	Stiff Inflexible	After urological surgery For bladder irrigation	Short-term use only
Latex	Made from purified rubber Soft	General use	Short-term use Causes urethral irritation Risk of latex allergy Prone to crust formation
Teflon-coated latex	PTFE coated Soft	General use	Short/medium-term use Reduced urethral trauma
Silicone elastomer	Silicone elastomer coated Reasonably soft	General use	Short/medium-term use Reduced encrustations
Pure silicone	Inert material Very soft Thin walled, larger lumen	Long-term catheterization	Long-term use Gradual deflation of balloon
Hydrogel coated	Soft Absorbs urethral mucosal secretions	Long-term catheterization	Long-term use Reduced encrustation Reduced bacterial colonisation
Narrow-lumen	Small calibre plastic catheters Stiff	For urodynamic testing	For immediate use
Intermittent	Made of PVC Hydrophilic Semi-stiff	Intermittent self- catheterization	Huge range of choice Usually single use

- Urine bypassing
- Catheter encrustation
- Social—embarrassment, impaired sexual function

(h) STANDARD SEMEN ANALYSIS

Overview
Infertility, defined by the inability of a couple to conceive after 1 year of unprotected intercourse, is relatively common.

- 20–25% of couples affected
- Male factor problems responsible in 50% of cases
- Semen analysis is the cornerstone of evaluation of the male partner

Semen analysis is highly indicative of the functional status of the testis by assessing the quantity, quality, and capabilities of semen in that particular specimen. Most men comply readily with semen analysis, but a small proportion of patients find masturbatory sample production distasteful and embarrassing and sensitivity is required when broaching the subject.

Indications
Infertility is the single most common indication for semen analysis, but a number of other indications exist:

- To ensure sterility after vasectomy
- For examination and/or storage if patient due to undergo fertility-threatening intervention (e.g., radiotherapy, orchidectomy)
- Prior to use for artificial insemination or cryopreservation
- Research—development of infertility treatments and new contraceptive methods

Technique
At least two samples (separated by a minimum of 1 week) are essential for diagnostic accuracy. The patient must be provided within clean (ideally sterile), wide-necked, dry, additive-free containers for specimen collection. Appropriate instructions must also be provided with regard to—

1. *Length of abstinence*: 2–3 days is ideal. A shorter period may result in abnormally lowered sperm counts, while a longer period of abstinence may result in a higher proportion of poorly motile sperms.

2. *Site of sample production*: providing the patient does not live more than 45 minutes away from the laboratory, the sample may be produced at home.

3. *Time of semen production*: samples produced and delivered in the morning allow maximal time for analytical tests.

4. *Method of sample production*: usually performed by masturbation but patient may chose to use coitus interruptus (risk of semen spillage) or non-toxic silastic condoms. Ordinary condoms contain rubber and spermicides which obliterate sperm motility.

5. *Transport of sample*: maintaining the sample at body temperature is ideal and excessive heating or cooling must be avoided.

Artifacts may arise due to—

• Low volume due to loss of semen due to spillage
• Contaminants (e.g., dust, fluff, soap, spermicidal crystals)
• Temperature variations (e.g., sunlight exposure or cooling in the fridge)

Interpretation

Normal values
Although a number of factors including period of abstinence, general health, stress, diet, medications, etc., can affect semen analysis, the World Health Organization has defined standard values (see Table 6.5).

TABLE 6.5. Semen analysis—standard values

Volume	1.5–5.0 ml
pH	7.0–8.0
Sperm concentration	≥20 million/mL
Total no. of spermatozoa	≥40 million/ejaculate
Motility	≥50% with progressive motility or 25% with rapid motility within 60 min after ejaculation
Morphology	≥50% normal shape and form by standard criteria, or ≥14% by strict criteria
Viability	≥50% of spermatozoa
Leukocytes	<1 million/mL

Other physical characteristics:

- The initially thick seminal coagulum usually liquefies within 5–30 min. Failure to liquefy within 1 hour of ejaculation is abnormal and may suggest infection, although in most cases is idiopathic

- Color
  - Normal semen is opalescent
  - Clear semen may be suggestive of a low sperm count
  - Pink or red semen is indicative of hematospermia and may in some circumstances warrant further investigation
  - Green semen is associated with infection and must be sent for microscopy and culture
  - Jaundice may result in orange discoloration of the semen due to excessive bilirubin in the semen

Abnormalities
The confirmation of two normal semen analyses, with no clearly identified risk factor in the history or physical examination of the male patient, should prompt evaluation of the female counterpart. Abnormal parameters may exist in isolation (uncommon) or in combination (more often); this is called oligo-astheno-teratozoospermia (OAT) syndrome. Some of the common abnormalities are described below:

Low volume
- Short period of abstinence
- Retrograde ejaculation (check urine for sperm)
- Infection (seminal vesiculitis, prostatitis)
- Obstruction (azospermia—ejaculatory duct obstruction, congenital absence of the vas)
- Endocrine disorder (check FSH, LH, and testosterone)

Variations in semen pH
- pH may become acidic in the presence of infection or congenital absence of vas

Low (oligospermia) or absent sperm (azospermia)
- Non-obstructive—varicoele, cryptorchidism (unilateral or bilateral), injury, illness, stress, or testicular failure
- Obstructive
  - Congenital—congenital absence of vas deferens (associated with cystic fibrosis)
  - Acquired—vasectomy or infection (e.g., epididymitis)

Poor motility (asthenospermia)
- Motility probably more important than sperm count
- Causes include prolonged abstinence, excessive heat (e.g., varicocoeles, hot baths), excessive alcohol, smoking, recreational drugs, toxin exposure (e.g., solvents, pesticides, lead, mercury, gold), urogenital infection, anti-sperm antibodies (e.g., after vasectomy or testicular trauma), partial ductal obstruction, and idiopathic

Increased abnormal morphology (teratozoospermia)
- Rarely occurs in isolation; causes include impaired spermatogenesis and testicular failure

In the absence of any abnormal parameters, if indicated, further adjunctive sperm function tests may be performed. These include—

- Computer-assisted semen analysis—to decrease subjective variables
- Seminal fructose testing—to detect seminal vesicle agenesis or obstruction
- Anti-sperm antibodies
- Semen leukocyte analysis—to detect an inflammatory etiology
- Sperm–cervical mucus interaction
- Sperm penetration assay—to assess the ability of sperm to penetrate a hamster egg
- Hypo-osmotic swelling test—to assess sperm motility

- Safe and non-invasive initial test for male factor sub-fertility
- If abnormal it suggests the likelihood of decreased fertility
- Prone to variations
- Not a direct measure of fertility
- Semen count and motility correlate best with fertility

(i) CYSTOSCOPY

Overview

Direct endoscopic visualization of the lower urinary tract still remains the gold standard procedure for the diagnosis of structural abnormalities in the bladder and urethra. Cystoscopy will allow demonstration of pathologies such as—

- Bladder tumors and stones
- Diverticula and scarring
- Urethral lesions (stones, strictures, prostatic occlusion)
- Provide access to the upper urinary tract

Cystoscopy requires an endoscope, camera head, irrigation, a light source, and a TV monitor (ideally with video recording facility).

Indications
- Investigation of hematuria
- Evaluation of troublesome LUTS which may be attributable to an intravesical or intra-urethral pathology
- Surveillance of bladder cancer
- Access for upper tract manipulation
- Diagnostic procedures (e.g., biopsy)
- Therapeutic procedures on the bladder (e.g., resection, urethral dilation, insertion of difficult catheter)

Technique
Patient preparation:

- Flexible cystoscopy—usually performed following intra-urethral instillation of 10 ml of 1% lidocaine-containing gel
- Rigid cystoscopy—requires either regional (e.g., spinal) or general anesthesia
- Due to the risk of UTI (up to 46%) and sepsis, high-risk patients (e.g., resection, presence of stone or urinary catheter, upper tract manipulation) must receive a single dose of prophylactic antibiotics (usually gentamicin or a quinolone)

Irrigation
The irrigation fluid may be—

- Conductive (contains electrolytes)—normal saline and Ringer's lactate solution
- Non-conductive—glycine and water allow electrocoagulation

In certain situations (e.g., visualization of the dome of bladder if view using irrigation fluid is suboptimal), an air cystoscopy may be useful.

TABLE 6.6. Features of rigid and flexible cystoscopes

	Rigid	Flexible
Components	Sheath Obturator Bridge Telescopes Working elements—(deflecting mechanism, biopsy forceps, etc.)	Fiber-optic light bearing bundle Fiber-optic image bearing bundle A single irrigation-working channel
Size	8–32F (8–12F for pediatric use)	14–17F
Lens	0°, 12°, 30°, 70°, 90°, and 120° lenses	0° lens only
Flexibility	None	Maximum deflection in one plane is 180–120°
Procedures	Biopsy Diathermy Resection Upper tract manipulation (e.g., ureteric catheterization or stent insertion) Lithoclast Bladder washout	Biopsy Electrocautery or laser ablation of small tumors Retrograde pyelography Insertion/removal of ureteric stents
Advantages	Better visualization due to superior optics Better irrigation flow Larger working channel Able to washout the bladder Manage large bladder tumors	Less discomfort Does not require sedation or anesthesia Can be performed supine Flexibility—better visualization of bladder neck
Disadvantages	Usually requires sedation, spinal, or general anesthesia Rigid—can miss bladder neck lesions Usually done in the dorsolithotomy position	Small working channel—biopsies may be inadequate Unable to wash bladder out View suboptimal if hematuria Unable to manage large bladder tumors

Type of instrument
The features of both rigid and flexible cystoscopes are discussed in the table above (Table 6.6).

Technique
- Inspection of the urethra requires a 0°, 12° or 30° telescope
- Careful attention must be paid to the following areas
  —the external urethral meatus
  —anterior (penile) urethra
  —external urethral sphincter
  —prostatic urethra (occlusion, length, vascularity)
  —bladder neck (open or tight/high)
- Upon entry into the bladder the residual urine volume is noted
- A systematic examination of the entire bladder is performed using either a 30° or 70° telescope, including—
  —state of the urothelium
  —degree of trabeculation
  —ureteric orifices
  —bladder neck (may require a 90° or 120° telescope if using a rigid instrument)
  —abnormalities (e.g., tumor, stones, diverticula, flat urothelial abnormalities)
- The bladder is emptied at the completion of the procedure

Complications
Complications can be significantly minimized by proper technique and avoiding cystoscopy in patients suspected of having an active UTI. The more frequent complications include—

- Dysuria (clears within 1 day)
- Hematuria (usually clears within 3 voids)
- UTI (<5% with prophylaxis, up to 38% without)
- Urethral trauma

Rarer complications include sepsis, bladder perforation, urethral false passage, and urethral stricture.

Part II

Urological Conditions Requiring Investigations

Chapter 7
Scrotal Pain and Swellings (Excluding Tumors)

OVERVIEW
- Patients with scrotal pain or swelling account for around 20% of all patients presenting to the urology clinic
- Scrotal pain is a common reason for hospital admission of boys
- Most scrotal masses can be diagnosed without formal investigation
- Defining the relationship of any scrotal lump to the testis proper is a cardinal feature in enabling correct diagnosis

(a) EPIDIDYMAL CYSTS
- Usually asymptomatic
- Benign, smooth, often spherical, fluctuant, and transilluminable cysts
- Distinctly palpated separate from the testis

Investigations (usually not required)
1. USS—may help confirm diagnosis in doubtful cases
2. needle aspiration—reveals straw-colored or opalescent fluid (sperm present)

(b) EPIDIDYMITIS
- Can affect males of any age
- Gradual onset scrotal pain, swelling, and erythema
- Some patients may complain of concurrent LUTS and fever
- A tender, swollen epididymis is the most common finding

Investigations
1. Urine dipstick—may suggest infection (leukocytes, nitrites)
2. MSU—to confirm infection
3. Urethral swab—to exclude chlamydia in the sexually active male

4. USS—may reveal a swollen epididymis; color Doppler may demonstrate increased blood flow; useful to confirm the absence of intratesticular malignancy. (Note: an anatomical or functional abnormality of the urinary tract is noted in 47–80% of prepubertal patients with a clinical diagnosis of epididymitis. Therefore USS of the entire urinary tract is mandatory in patients within this age group (± micturating cystourethrography)

Additional investigations
1. Serum tumor markers—AFP, βHCG, and LDH if concerned about a malignant differential diagnosis
2. EMU (×3)—for detection of *Mycobacterium* tuberculosis
3. TRUS—to exclude anatomical abnormality of the seminal vesicles

---

(c) SCROTAL ABSCESS
- May arise as a complication of untreated epididymo-orchitis or secondary to scrotal skin pathology (e.g., infected sebaceous cyst)
- Acutely tender, swollen, erythematous, and fluctuant scrotum
- Pus discharge may be obvious
- Patient may be systemically unwell
- Diagnosis primarily based on clinical findings

Investigations
1. US scan—may reveal abscess cavity and local vascularity
2. Urine dipstick
3. MSU
4. Blood cultures
5. Culture of aspirated or drained cavity contents

(d) TESTICULAR TORSION
- Represents a true urological emergency
- History and physical examination is paramount
- Scrotal exploration should ideally be undertaken within 6 hours from onset of pain to minimise the risk of testicular ischemia

Investigations
1. Scrotal exploration—if sufficiently concerned, surgery is the only investigation (and therapeutic procedure) required. This is performed under general anesthesia and final outcomes include—

- Orchidopexy
- Orchidectomy (if testis non-viable)
- Contralateral orchidopexy if true torted testis

2. Doppler US scan—not indicated in the diagnosis of torsion (due to significant false-positive and false-negative results), but more useful for confirmation of absence of torsion if surgery not deemed necessary. Doppler techniques will demonstrate normal testicular blood supply.

3. Radionuclide imaging is useful in the evaluation of testicular blood flow but is time-consuming and relatively inaccurate for the diagnosis of acute torsion.

(e) HYDROCELE
- May be confined to the scrotum or may extend in to inguinal ring (associated with a hernia)
- Diagnosis usually apparent on clinical examination

Investigations
1. MSU—to exclude underlying infection
2. USS—to ensure healthy underlying testis (as 10% of hydroceles are secondary to testicular infection, tumor or trauma)

(f) VARICOCELE
- Predominantly left-sided varicosities of the pampiniform plexus veins
- Diagnosis and grading based on clinical findings
  - Grade I   palpable only with valsalva maneuver
  - Grade II   palpable in standing position
  - Grade III visible through scrotal skin

Investigations
1. Doppler USS—can confirm diagnosis and grading. All grade III varicoceles should undergo USS of the retroperitoneum to exclude obstruction of the testicular vein (e.g., from a renal tumor, retroperitoneal nodes).

2. Venography—in some centers, venography is preferred for demonstration of varicocele anatomy. This has been the traditional gold standard investigation, but due to its invasive nature (requires access through either the common femoral or internal jugular vein), it has been superseded by USS.

Chapter 8
Lower Urinary Tract Symptoms (LUTS)

OVERVIEW

A wide range of conditions produce apparently similar LUTS (see Table 8.1). The majority of patients presenting to the urology clinic complain of LUTS. Even experienced urologists therefore rely on investigations for accurate diagnosis.

(i) BLADDER OUTLET OBSTRUCTION
- Common causes
  - Benign prostatic obstruction (symptomatic, retention of urine)
  - Bladder neck obstruction
  - Urethral stricture

- Symptoms
  - Typically, symptoms of flow disturbance (e.g., hesitancy, poor, prolonged, or intermittent flow) dominate over irritative (frequency, urgency, and urge incontinence) symptoms
  - Retention of urine
    ◊ Acute or acute on chronic retention (painful)
  - Chronic retention is usually painless—residual urine usually >1 liter

  (Tip: history of incontinence [including bed wetting] in the presence of a palpable bladder should alert the clinician to the possibility of high-pressure chronic retention with the attending risk of upper tract dilatation and renal failure)

  In cases of doubt a bedside bladder scan gives an estimate of residual urine.

  (Tip: if insertion of a supra-pubic catheter is contemplated, it is always safer to obtain a bladder scan prior to insertion)

- **Minimal set of investigations**
  - Digital rectal examination of prostate
  - Estimation of serum creatinine (to assess renal function)

- FVC (filled for at least 3 days)
- I-PSS or AUA symptom score assessment (see Table 8.2)
- MSSU
- Urine flow rate
- Post-void bladder residual urine estimation

- **Recommended investigations** (if history of infection, urothelial tumor, urinary stones, infection or retention)
  - USS of upper urinary tract
  - KUB—to exclude radio-opaque calculi
  - Flexible cystoscopy—to exclude a urethral stricture or an intravesical lesion

- **Additional investigations (if diagnosis uncertain or confirmation needed)**
  - Urodynamic studies—conventional or video cystometry to investigate BOO in the following patient categories (*EAU guidelines on treatment of BPH*)
    —Men <50 years of age or >80 years of age
    —Post void residual urine >300 mL
    —Suspicion of neurogenic bladder dysfunction
    —Previous radical pelvic surgery
    —Previous surgery for relief of bladder outlet obstruction
    —Suspected detrusor overactivity

  - Investigations to evaluate urethral strictures
    —Urethrogram
    —Ultrasound scan of urethra
    —MR scan of penis to evaluate urethra and peri-urethral structures

---

(ii) URINARY INCONTINENCE

(a) Stress
- Symptoms
  - Leakage when patient coughs, sneezes, runs, or lifts heavy objects
  - Insensible loss
  - Recurrent UTIs

(Tip: during each episode the amount of urine leakage due to stress incontinence is usually small. If patient says that the leakage is large [as if the bladder is emptying itself] suspect concurrent detrusor overactivity)

- **Minimal set of investigations**
  - MSSU
  - FVC

- **Recommended investigations**
  - Pad test—to estimate degree of wetness
  - Urodynamic studies—ideally videourodynamics (particularly prior to surgical intervention or if associated urge symptoms)

(b) Urge
- Symptoms
  - Urine leakage associated with urgency
  - Frequency, nocturia

- **Minimal set of investigations**
  - MSSU
  - FVC
  - Bladder residual urine volume estimation

- **Recommended investigations**
  - Urodynamic studies—to confirm detrusor overactivity
  - Flexible cystoscopy—to exclude an intravesical lesion (tumor, CIS) in all patients >40 years of age with irritative symptoms

(c) Lower urinary tract fistulae
- Types
  - Vesico-vaginal
  - Uretero-vaginal
  - Urethro-vaginal
  - Urethro-rectal
  - Colo-vesical

- **Investigations (depends on location of fistulae)**
  - IVU—to exclude ureteric involvement
  - Cystogram—especially CT cystogram
  - Cystoscopy and (swab test if needed)
  - CT or MRI (especially useful in colo-vesical fistula)

(iii) LOWER URINARY TRACT INFECTIONS

- **Minimal set of investigations** (if solitary UTI in a female)
  - MSSU

- **Recommended investigation** (if recurrent UTIs; UTI in male patients; or upper tract involvement—pyelonephritis)
  - Flow rate and post void residual urine volume estimation (especially in men)
  - KUB—to exclude renal tract calculi
  - USS—of upper urinary tract
  - Flexible cystoscopy (in intractable cases)—may also be therapeutic in case of recurrent urethritis/urethral syndrome in women
  - If prostatitis suspected:
    - ◊ Expressed prostatic secretions for microscopy and culture
    - ◊ Semen microscopy and culture
    - ◊ Fractional urine specimens for microscopy and culture
    - ◊ Urethral swab or urine specimen for detection of *Chlamydia trachomatis*

(iv) CHRONIC PELVIC PAIN SYNDROME/INTERSTITIAL CYSTITIS

- Defined as non-malignant pain perceived in structures related to the pelvis
- Urological syndromes include: (only the first two will be discussed in this section)
  - Painful bladder syndrome/interstitial cystitis
  - Prostate pain syndrome
  - Urethral pain syndrome
  - Chronic orchalgia

(a) Chronic Bladder Pain/Interstitial Cystitis (IC)

- Etiology unknown
- Patients describe pain, frequency, and nocturia
- Diagnosis based on symptoms, examination, urinary investigation and cystoscopy
- List of automatic exclusions include—
  - Age <18 year of age
  - Lower urinary tract or gynaecological tumors
  - Cystitis (bacterial, tuberculous, radiation, drug-induced) or vaginitis
  - Bladder or lower ureteric stones
  - Frequency of <5 times in 12 hours
  - Nocturia <twice
  - Duration <12 months
  - Bladder capacity >400 mL
  - Detrusor overactivity on UDS

- **Minimal set of investigations (if painful bladder syndrome suspected)**
  - Urine dipstick
  - MSSU – to exclude infection
  - EMU (×3)—for detection of *Mycobacterium tuberculosis*
  - FVC
  - Urodynamics—filling and voiding cystometry
    ◊ Measure bladder capacity
    ◊ Confirm reduced bladder compliance
    ◊ Exclude detrusor overactivity
  - Cystoscopy and biopsy
    ◊ Hunner's ulcer confirms diagnosis of IC
    ◊ Glomerulations (petechial hemorrhages) is very suggestive of IC
    ◊ Biopsies may support diagnosis of IC (and help exclude CIS)

(b) Prostate Pain Syndrome/Prostatitis

- Four types of prostatitis recognized:
  - Acute bacterial
  - Chronic bacterial
  - Chronic pelvic pain syndrome
    ◊ A: inflammatory—WBC in semen/EPS/VB3 urine
    ◊ B: non-inflammatory—no WBC in semen/EPS/VB3 urine
  - Asymptomatic inflammatory prostatitis (histological prostatitis)

- **Minimal set of investigations (if prostatitis suspected)**
  - Urine dipstick
  - MSSU
  - EPS
  - VB3 urine analysis
  - Semen culture and microscopy
  - Chlamydia serology

- **Additional recommended investigation**
  - TRUS (to exclude structural abnormalities)
  - Cystoscopy (to exclude urethral or intravesical lesions)
  - MR scan pelvis

TABLE 8.1. LUTS and conditions

LUTS	Condition Producing Symptoms
Frequency of voiding	
Frequency	Lower tract infections
	BOO
	Detrusor overactivity
	Foreign body in bladder (including ureteric stent)
	↓ bladder capacity (e.g., interstitial cystitis, post-radiation)
	Habitual
Nocturia	Excessive fluid intake
	BOO
	Detrusor overactivity
	Nocturnal polyuria (>30% of daily urine production occurs at nighttime hours)
Double micturition	Chronic retention of urine
	Large bladder diverticulum
	Severe VUR
Urgency	
Sensory urgency	Cystitis
	Carcinoma in situ
	Small bladder capacity
	Habitual
	BOO
Incontinence	
Stress	Genuine stress incontinence
	External urethral sphincter weakness (e.g., post-prostatectomy)
Urge	Detrusor overactivity
	Neurogenic bladder
	BOO
Overflow	Chronic (high pressure) retention of urine
Bed wetting	Primary nocturnal enuresis
	Chronic high pressure retention
	Excessive alcohol consumption at night
	Stress incontinence
	Severe sphincter weakness
Continuous (insensible)	Vesico-vaginal fistula
	Severe sphincter weakness

TABLE 8.1. *Continued*

LUTS	Condition Producing Symptoms
Post-micturition dribbling	BOO Urethral stricture Incomplete emptying of urethra

Incomplete bladder emptying	Lower urinary tract infections
	Chronic retention of urine
	Large bladder diverticulum
	Severe VUR
	(in the latter two due to
	    accumulation of false residual
	    urine in the bladder)

Sensory symptoms "Pressure down below"	Urethritis (urethral syndrome) Lower tract infections Atrophic vaginitis Chronic pelvic pain syndrome
Suprapubic pain	Lower urinary tract infections (prostatitis) Chronic pelvic pain syndrome Acute retention of urine Interstitial cystitis
Pain during micturition	Lower urinary tract infections (urethritis, prostatitis) Interstitial cystitis Urethral stricture Impacted urethral stone
Flow disturbances Hesitancy	BOO Detrusor sphincter/bladder neck dyssynergia Hypotonic detrusor Anxious bladder syndrome (anxiety)
Poor flow	BOO Hypotonic detrusor
Intermittent flow	BOO Anxiety

Inability to void	Urinary retention (due to BOO,
	    detrusor failure, anxiety,
	    constipation, drugs,
	    anesthesia, etc.)

Straining to pass urine	BOO Hypotonic detrusor

Over the Past Month or So	Not at all	Less than one time in 5	Less than half the time	About half the time	More than half the time	Almost always
How often have you had a sensation of not emptying your bladder after you finished urinating?	0	1	2	3	4	5
How often have you had to urinate again less than 2 hours after you finished urinating?	0	1	2	3	4	5
How often have you found you stopped and started again several times when you urinated?	0	1	2	3	4	5
How often have you found it difficult to postpone urination?	0	1	2	3	4	5
How often have you had a weak urinary stream?	0	1	2	3	4	5
How often have you had to push or strain to begin urination?	0	1	2	3	4	5
How many times did you most typically get up to urinate from the time you went to bed at night until you got up in the morning?	0	1	2	3	4	5

Total IPSS score = (out of 35)

- <7 mild symptoms
- 8–19 moderate symptoms
- >20 severe symptoms

Quality of life due to urinary symptoms:
If you were to spend the rest of your life with your urinary condition just the way it is now, how would you feel about that?

0 = delighted
1 = pleased
2 = mostly satisfied
3 = mixed (equally satisfied and dissatisfied)
4 = mostly dissatisfied
5 = unhappy
6 = terrible

Chapter 9
Loin Pain

OVERVIEW
- Loin pain may be caused by—
  - Renal calculi
  - Ureteral calculi
  - Urinary tract obstruction
  - Urinary tract infection
- Type, severity, and location of the pain may vary due to the size, location, degree, and acuity of obstruction or infection
- Loin pain may be atypical in nature and renal colic can be mistaken for other conditions
- The history, physical examination, and radiological imaging are essential to establish the correct diagnosis

---

(i) URINARY STONES

Symptoms are varied and may include—

- Acute renal or ureteral colic—the classic symptoms include colicky flank pain with radiation to the groin, ipsilateral testicle, or labia
- Mild abdominal or flank discomfort
- Nausea and vomiting
- Hematuria (microscopic or gross)
- UTI
- High-grade fevers or sepsis may ensue
- Irritative LUTS—distal ureteric stones may present with frequency, urgency, and dysuria

Which investigation for stones?

KUB
- Helpful in documenting the number, size, and location of stones
- Radiopacity may provide information regarding stones type

- Will identify calcium stones >1–2 mm in diameter
- Will miss most uric acid and some cystine calculi
- Will identify nephrocalcinosis—seen in hyperparathyroidism, primary hyperoxaluria, renal tubular acidosis, or sarcoidosis

Ultrasound
- Useful as a screening tool for hydronephrosis or stones within the kidney or renal pelvis
- Provides information on renal parenchyma in an obstructed kidney
- May detect radiolucent calculi
- Useful to rule out other causes of abdominal pain
- Middle and distal ureter are not clearly visible
- Useful for follow-up evaluation in recurrent nephrolithiasis

Intravenous urography
- Often the only test required for making management decisions in stone patients
- Can be performed by a non-radiologist in an emergency
- Provides precise information on the relationship of the calculus to the pelvicalyceal system and the ureter

Computed tomography
- Helical CT more sensitive than KUB, IVU, or USS
- Will detect radiolucent calculi
- Other conditions that mimic ureteral colic can be easily identified
- May be useful in determining some composition
- Poor detection of Indinavir stones

Current recommendations
- Non-contrast helical CT is the imaging study of choice to evaluate patients with suspected stone disease, in the acute setting (emergency department)
- If known history of nephrolithiasis is present, a KUB, USS, or both may provide initial low-cost confirmation of a recurrent stone that requires further radiographic evaluation

(a) Acute ureteric colic
- Caused by acute urinary obstruction with subsequent distention of the collecting system or ureter
- Type, severity, and location of the pain may vary due to the size, location, degree, and acuity of obstruction caused by the stones
- Renal colic can be mistaken for other conditions

- **Minimal set of investigations**
  1. Urine dipstick—reveals either microscopic or gross hematuria
  2. MSSU—mild pyuria may be associated with concurrent stones even in the absence of a UTI
  3. Serum creatinine
  4. KUB

- **Recommended investigations:**
  5. CT scan (non-contrast helical)
  6. IVU

- **Additional investigations:**
  7. USS—to assess hydronephrosis

(b) Renal stones
- Symptoms may be similar to those of acute ureteric colic, but commonly are related to a dull ache in the loin radiating anteriorly towards the abdomen
- Hematuria—microscopic or gross
- Symptoms may mimic appendicitis, cholecystitis, peptic ulcer disease, pancreatitis, ectopic pregnancy, or dissecting aortic aneurysm
- Costovertebral angle tenderness

- **Investigations (as for acute ureteric colic)**
  1. Urine dipstick
  2. MSSU
  3. Serum creatinine
  4. KUB
  5. USS
  6. IVU
  7. CT scan (non-contrast helical)

- **Additional investigations**
  8. Radionucleotide study (renography)—to assess relative renal function

(c) Bladder stones
- Presents with LUTS—frequency, urgency, hesitancy and dysuria
- Dysuria may radiate to the labia or tip of the penis
- Gross hematuria
- Physical examination findings usually non-specific

- **Minimal investigations**
  1. Urine dipstick—hematuria and leukocytosis usually present
  2. Cystoscopy—is both diagnostic and therapeutic (cystolitholopaxy)

- **Additional investigation** (these will detect the bladder calculi but ultimately cystoscopy will be required for treatment)
  3. USS
  4. KUB
  5. CT scan

(d) Stones in continent pouch
- Symptoms usually vague with mild abdominal discomfort
- Possible signs of urinary tract infection
- Hematuria
- Pyuria from the continent pouch
- Physical examination findings are non-specific

- **Investigations**
  1. MSSU
  2. KUB
  3. CT scan (non-contrast helical)

(ii) UPPER URINARY TRACT OBSTRUCTION

- Symptoms may be similar to renal or ureteral calculi
- Symptoms based on the acuteness of obstruction
- Urinary tract infection or mild abdominal/loin discomfort often present
- High-grade fevers or sepsis may ensue, due to the chronicity of the obstruction
- Hematuria is rarely seen
- Typically have loin pain after diuresis (drinking caffeinated beverages or alcohol)
- Nausea and vomiting are common

(a) Ureteropelvic junction obstruction (UPJO)
- Classically identified in young women (age 20–40)
- Type, severity, and location of the pain may vary
- Usually present with a dull ache in the loin worsened after drinking fluids
- Loin pain may be atypical in nature—often mistaken for other non-renal pain

- Associated nausea and emesis
- Costovertebral angle tenderness on examination

- **Investigations**
  1. Urine dipstick—usually will be normal
  2. MSSU
  3. USS—to assess hydronephrosis but not accurate for diagnosing UPJO
  4. IVU—may help determine degree of obstruction and suggests impairment of renal function
  5. CT scan—will demonstrate hydronephrosis and assess amount of remaining renal parenchyma
  6. Radionucleotide diuresis renography—will precisely determine degree of UPJO and/or renal impairment
  7. Retrograde pyelogram demonstrates exact location and extent of UPJO

(b) Ureteric obstruction (stricture/tumor)
- Signs and symptoms vary but similar to those seen in UPJO

- **Investigations**
  1. Urine dipstick
  2. MSSU
  3. Urine cytology—may be positive in cases of ureteral tumor
  4. USS
  5. IVU
  6. CT scan
  7. Diuresis renography
  8. Retrograde pyelogram demonstrates exact location and extent of ureteral stricture or tumor

(c) Vesico-ureteric reflux
- VUR is discussed later in the book with primary reference to vesico-ureteric reflux in children (see Chapter 5a)

(iii) UPPER URINARY TRACT INFECTIONS

- Combination of flank pain and fever constitutes a potentially dangerous symptomatology
- Sepsis may ensue
- Hematuria (microscopic or gross) is commonly seen, along with signs of urinary tract infection
- With documented urinary tract infection and obstruction, antibiotics alone is not sufficient treatment—the collecting system must be decompressed

- **Investigations**
  1. Urine dipstick—may reveal hematuria and pyuria
  2. MSSU—to identify the uro-pathogen
  3. Serum electrolytes
  4. Full blood count
  5. Blood cultures
  6. KUB
  7. USS—to assess hydronephrosis but not accurate for the exact diagnosis of pyelonephritis
  8. IVU—to exclude obstruction secondary to stone
  9. CT scan

Chapter 10
Urological Cancers

HEMATURIA
- A common urological condition
- If heavy, hospitalization may be required
- Three types:
  1. Macroscopic
  2. Microscopic
  3. Dipstix (lab stick)
- In most patients >40 years of age, further investigations are mandatory
- A urinary tract abnormality is found in >20% of the cases (see Table 10.1)
- Urological cancers may present as hematuria

Minimal set of investigations
For microscopic & dipstix hematuria

1. MSSU
2. Serum electrolytes and creatinine
3. KUB
4. USS
5. Consider referral to nephrologist (may require renal biopsy?)
6. Cytological examination of urine
7. Cystoscopy

For macroscopic hematuria

1. MSSU
2. Urine cytology
3. Serum electrolytes and creatinine
4. USS
5. IVU or CT scan
6. Cystoscopy
7. Upper tract endoscopy

TABLE 10.1. Causes of hematuria

Renal

Stones
Renal tumor (e.g., Renal cell carcinoma)
Transitional cell carcinoma
Papillary necrosis
Tuberculosis
Pyelonephritis
Parenchymal disease (glomerulonephritis, nephropathy)

Ureter

Stones
Transitional cell carcinoma

Bladder and prostate

Transitional cell carcinoma
Stones
Bacterial cystitis
Tuberculosis
Radiation cystitis
Interstitial cystitis
Schisotomiosis
Benign prostatic hyperplasia

Urethra

Urethritis
Stone
Tumor
Stricture

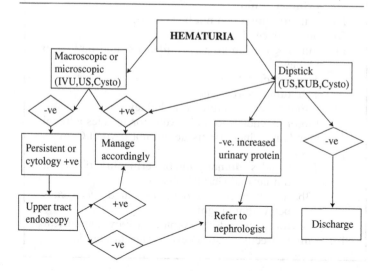

(a) RENAL

- Most solid tumors of the kidney are malignant
- Most common tumor is renal cell carcinoma (RCC—also referred to as hypernephroma or adenocarcinoma of the kidney)

- Presentation
    - Incidental finding(>60% of the tumors)
    - Hematuria
    - Loin pain
    - Loin mass
    - Anemia
    - Weight loss
    - Acute abdominal pain
    - Hypovolemic shock (due to retroperitoneal bleeding—not uncommon with angio-myo-lipoma)
    - Paraneoplastic syndromes (noted in up to 10% of tumors)

- Solid tumors of the kidney
    - RCC
    - Oncocytoma
    - Angiomyolipoma

- TNM classification of renal cell carcinoma

T: primary tumor
TX: primary tumor can not be assessed
T0: no evidence of primary tumor
T1: tumor < 7 cm in greatest dimension and limited to kidney
    T1a: tumor < 4 cm
    T1b: tumor > 4 cm and <7 cm
T2: tumor > 7 cm and limited to kidney
T3: tumor extends into major veins or invades adrenal gland or perinephric tissue but not beyond Gerota's fascia
    T3a: invades adrenal gland or perinephric tissue but not beyond Gerota's fascia
    T3b: tumor extends into renal vein or vena cava below diaphragm
    T3c: tumor extends into vena cava above diaphragm
T4: tumor directly invades beyond Gerota's fascia

> **N: regional lymph nodes**
> Nx: status can not be assessed
> N0: no regional lymph nodes
> N1: single regional lymph node
> N2: more than one regional lymph node
>
> **M: distant metastasis**
> Mx: metastasis cannot be assessed
> M0: no metastasis
> M1: distant metastasis

Investigations if tumor suspected

- Blood tests
  - Full hematological profile
  - Urea and electrolytes
  - Liver function tests
  - Bone profile (including serum calcium)
- USS
- CT scan (pre and post contrast to assess enhancement)
- Chest X-ray or CT scan of lung
- Consider bone scan—if bone pain or hypercalcemia

Renal cysts

- Usually incidental findings
- If simple (type I)—no further investigations needed
- If complex (type II or greater)—pre- and post-contrast CT scan is mandatory
- Risk of malignancy in Type III and IV is high (40–100%)
- Classified according to Bosniak:
  - Type I: simple cyst, no septa, no calcification
  - Type II: cyst with thin septa, no or fine calcification in the wall, wall/s do not enhance on post-contrast CT
  - Type IIF: Minimal thickening of septa or wall, coarse calcification, no enhancing soft tissue elements
  - Type III: more like cystic masses, thick irregular walls or septa which enhance
  - Type IV: abnormalities are more obvious than in Type III with more enhancing soft tissue lesions

(b) ADRENAL

Investigations if tumor suspected

- Urinary adrenal markers (see Chapter 1e—Urinary Adrenal Markers)
- Serum adrenal markers (see Chapter 2f—Serum Markers of Adrenal Function)
- CT scan (pre- and post-contrast) or MR scan
  - CT can differentiate between benign and malignant tumors based on—
    - ◊ Density (Hounsfield units)
      - ✦ <10 benign adenoma
      - ✦ 10–30 equivivocal
      - ✦ >30 malignant
    - ◊ Washout of contrast from the tumor
      - ✦ Pre-contrast CT is performed
      - ✦ Administration of IV contrast
      - ✦ Delayed scan performed after 2 minutes
      - ✦ If >50% contrast washout it is less likely to be malignant
    - ◊ Other features: size (>3 cm, presence of calcification, irregular edges—all increase the possibility of malignancy)

(c) UROTHELIAL

- TCC is the most common urothelial tumor
- Squamous cell carcinoma of the bladder is more common in some parts of the world (e.g., Middle East, North Africa)
- TNM classification of bladder tumors

T:	**primary tumor**
Ta:	non-invasive papillary tumor
Tis	(cis): carcinoma in situ
T1:	involving sub-epithelial connective tissue
T2:	involving muscularis propria
	T2a: superficial
	T2b: deep
T3:	beyond muscularis propria and into perivesical fat
	T3a: microscopically
	T3b: extravesical mass

T4: Tumor involving prostate, uterus, vagina, pelvic
     wall, or abdominal wall
     T4a: prostate, uterus or vagina
     T4b: pelvic wall or abdominal wall

N: regional lymph nodes
N1: single node <2 cm
N2: single 2–5 cm, multiple <5 cm each
N3: >5 cm

Investigations if bladder tumor suspected
- MSSU
- Urine cytology
- IVU OR CT urogram
- Cystoscopy
- Consider MR scan (if invasive tumor is suspected)

Investigations if upper tract tumor suspected
- MSSU
- Urine cytology
- IVU or CT urogram
- Retrograde ureterogram (not as reliable as endoscopy)
- Upper tract endoscopy (uretero-pyeloscopy)
- Please note:
  - Larger exophytic tumors may be seen with above imaging studies
  - Tumors located at the bladder base may be difficult to differentiate from an intra-vesical prostate growth (benign or malignant)
  - CT and/or MR can help stage urothelial tumors (but post-resection edema may be confused with invasive disease on CT/MR scanning)
  - The imaging modalities are diagnostic aids only and endoscopic confirmation of the diagnosis is required

(d) PROSTATE
- Most common male cancer
- Increased male life expectancy and PSA screening program is resulting in a rapid increase in incidence

- May or may not present with symptoms (LUTS, bone pain from metastatic disease)
- TNM classification of prostate cancer

T: primary tumor
Tx: primary tumor can not be assessed
T0:   no evidence of primary tumor
T1:   clinically not palpable or not visible on imaging
     T1a: incidental histological finding <5% of resected tissue
     T1b: incidental finding in >5% of resected tissue
     T1c: identified on needle biopsy—because of elevated serum PSA level
T2:   Tumor confined to prostate
     T2a: involving one lobe
     T2b: involving both lobes
T3:   tumor extends through prostate capsule
     T3a: unilateral or bilateral extension
     T3b: involving seminal vesicle/s
T4:   tumor invading adjacent structures other than seminal vesicles (bladder neck; external sphincter, rectum, pelvic floor muscles, pelvic wall)

N: regional lymph nodes
Nx: regional lymph node status can not be assessed
N0:   no regional lymph node metastasis
N1:   regional lymph node metastasis present

M: distant metastases
Mx: not assessed
M0:   no metastasis
M1:   distant metastasis
     M1a: non-regional lymph node/s
     M1b: bone metastasis
     M1c: other sites

Investigations if prostate cancer suspected
- Digital rectal examination
- PSA (see Chapter 2a—PSA)
- TRUS and prosate biopsy (see Chapter 6a—TRUS)
- MRI (useful for staging once diagnosis confirmed)
- Bone scan (for evidence of metastatic disease)

(e) PENIS

- Squamous cell carcinoma is the most common type
- Several pre-malignant conditions including balanitis xerotica obliterans, leukoplakia, penile cutaneous horn, condyloma acuminate, penile carcinoma in situ (Bowen's disease, erythroplasia of Queyrat, and bowenoid papulosis)
- TNM classification of penile tumors

T: primary tumor
Tx: primary tumor can not be assessed
T0: no primary tumor
Tis: carcinoma in situ
Ta: non-invasive verrrucous carcinoma
T1: invasion of subepithelial connective tissue
T2: invasion of corpus spongiosum or cavernosum
T3: invasion of urethra or prostate
T4: invasion of adjacent structures

N: regional lymph nodes
Nx: lymph node status cannot be assessed
N0: no lymph nodal involvement
N1: metastasis in one inguinal node
N2: metastasis in multiple or bilateral superficial inguinal nodes
N3: metastasis in deep inguinal or pelvic nodes

M: distant metastases
Mx: distant metastasis cannot be assessed
M0: no distant metastasis
M1: distant metastasis present

Investigations if penile cancer suspected
- Clinical examination (penis and inguinal region)
- USS or MR scan of the penis (may help evaluate local invasion)
- CT or MR scan of abdomen and pelvis (for staging)
- Bone scan (if bone metastasis suspected)
- Biopsy of lesion or circumcision for histological confirmation
- Note: imaging studies are useful but histological diagnosis is mandatory

(f) TESTIS

- Usually present as painless scrotal lump
- Primary tumors common in young men
- Lymphoma common in older men
- Classification of tumors

Germ cell tumors
Intratubular germ cell neoplasia
Seminoma
Embryonal carcinoma
Yolk sac tumor
Chorio-carcinoma
Teratoma
Mixed

Sex cord stromal tumors
Leydig cell tumor
Sertoli cell tumor
Granulosa
Mixed

Mixed germ cell and sex cord tumors

TNM classification of testicular tumors

T:	**primary tumor**
Tx:	tumor cannot be assessed
T0:	no primary tumor
Tis:	carcinoma in situ
T1:	tumor limited to testis and epididymis without vascular or lymphatic invasion (tumor may invade tunica albuginia but not vaginalis)
T2:	tumor limited to testis and epididymis + vascular or lymphatic invasion or invasion of tunica vaginalis
T3:	tumor invades spermatic cord (with or without vascular or lymphatic invasion)
T4:	tumor invades scrotum with or without vascular or lymphatic invasion

N: **regional lymph nodes**
Nx: lymph node status cannot be assessed
N0: no lymph node metastasis
N1: single or multiple <2 cm in greatest dimension
N2: nodes 2–5 cm in greatest dimension
N3: nodes >5 cm in greatest dimension

M: **distant metastases**
Mx: distant metastasis cannot be assessed
M0: no distant metastasis
M1: distant metastasis present
   M1a: non-regional nodes or lung
   M1b: other sites

Investigations if testicular cancer suspected

- Clinical examination of testes and supraclavicular nodes
- Serum tumor markers (see Chapter 2c—Testicular Tumor Markers)
- USS (including Doppler interrogation)
- CT scan (chest, abdomen and pelvis to assess lymph node status)
- Bone scan (if bone metastasis suspected)
- Ultimately, orchidectomy will establish histological diagnosis

Chapter 11
Congenital and Pediatric Disorders

(a) HYDRONEPHROSIS

Overview
- Hydronephrosis is not a diagnosis in itself, but merely a description of dilatation of the collecting system
- Detectable early within the prenatal period (from week 16) and in most instances will resolve within 1 week of birth
- May be unilateral or bilateral
- May be acute or chronic (often associated with thinning of renal cortex)
- May be seen in conjunction with dilatation of the ureters (hydroureteronephrosis)

The commonest causes of hydronephrosis in the pediatric population are—

- Ureteropelvic junction obstruction (UPJO)
- Vesico-ureteric reflux (VUR)
- Megaureters
- Urethral valve syndrome
- Multicystic renal dysplasia

UPJO
- Accounts for about half of all hydronephrosis in children
- Incidence of 1:1,000
- Males affected as commonly as females
- About 20% eventually undergo surgical correction (pyeloplasty)
- Etiology of the obstruction may be intrinsic or extrinsic (crossing lower pole vessels)
- The usual modes of presentation are—
  - Incidental finding
  - UTI

- Pain—abdominal or loin
- Hematuria
- Abdominal mass

VUR

- Retrograde flow of urine from the bladder into the upper urinary tract
- Prevalence between 1% and 2% of the general pediatric population
- More common in girls compared to boys till the age of 1 year, and then this relationship is reversed
- Males more likely to present symptomatically during the first year of life, while females present later (2–7 years)
- Hydronephrosis seen twice as often in boys as in girls
- Causes of VUR are classified as—
  - Primary—anatomical abnormality resulting in incompetent vesico-ureteric junction (genetic predisposition)
  - Secondary—to neuropathic bladders, PUV, ureteric duplication, detrusor overactivity

The significance of VUR lies in the fact that between 25% and 40% of such patients show demonstrable evidence of renal scarring (due to a combination of intra-renal reflux and infection) at first presentation. Renal scarring may lead to hypertension and end-stage renal failure. Surveillance is therefore essential. VUR may present as—

- UTI (30%)
- Renal failure
- Hypertension
- Urinary incontinence

VUR is classified using the International Reflux Study Committee classification (Fig 11.1):

- Grade I—into ureter only
- Grade II—reflux into renal pelvis but no dilatation
- Grade III—as grade II but with mild to moderate dilatation of the pelvicalyceal system, minimal blunting
- Grade IV—as grade III but with moderate dilatation
- Grade V—gross dilatation of the collecting system and ureteric tortuosity

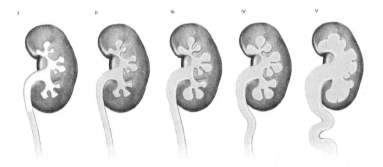

FIGURE 11.1. Classification of VUR

Minimal set of investigations (for UPJO or VUR)
1. Urine dipstick
2. MSSU
3. Renal function assessment—serum creatinine estimation or more sophisticated techniques of renal function estimation (e.g., creatinine clearance)
4. USS—will demonstrate kidney size, thickness of the paren-chyma, cortical echo-pattern, AP diameter of renal pelvis, calyceal ectasia, width of ureter, bladder wall thickness, and residual urine
5. MCUG—will confirm presence of VUR and allow grading. Also useful for evaluation of urethral valves
6. Static (DMSA) renal scintigraphy—ideal method for assess-ment of renal cortical morphology, infection changes, renal scars, and relative function estimation (avoid in the first 2 months of life)
7. Diuresis (MAG3) renography—to distinguish between obstruc-tive and non-obstructive causes of hydronephrosis, and calcu-lation of split renal function

Additional investigations
1. *IVU*—may be useful to demonstrate the anatomy if surgery is being considered
2. *Whitaker's test*—only considered if diagnosis of obstruction is suspected but not proven on diuresis renography
3. Cystoscopy—may be of some use if the entire lower urinary tract has not satisfactorily been visualised on MCUG. Also allows assessment of site, size, number and morphology of the ureteric orifice.

(b) URINARY TRACT INFECTION (UTI)

Overview

- The urinary tract is a common source of infection in the pediatric population
- 4% of girls and 1% of boys will have a UTI before puberty
- 50% of girls with one UTI will have a further infection
- *E. coli* is responsible for around 85% of UTI in children
- Mechanisms of pathogen entry include—
  - Retrograde ascent of perineal bacteria (most common)
  - Following instrumentation of the urinary tract
  - Involvement of the urinary tract as part of systemic infection

The significance of pediatric UTI is that between 30% and 50% are associated with a urinary tract anomaly and 15–30% demonstrate evidence of renal scarring at initial presentation. An anatomical or functional abnormality is more likely the younger the patient is at first presentation. Urinary tract investigations are mandatory, especially in patients before the age of 4 due to the increased susceptibility of the kidneys to undergo scarring. Common associations noted in patients with UTI include—

- VUR (about 50%)
- UPJO
- Vesico-ureteric junction obstruction
- Ureteroceles
- Duplication anomalies

UTI in children is classified as—

- Asymptomatic bacteriuria—significant bacteriuria on MSU analysis but without any symptoms
- Cystitis—irritative symptoms related to bladder involvement, no systemic symptoms or fever
- Acute pyelonephritis—febrile infection of the renal parenchyma
- Complicated UTI—secondary to anatomical or functional abnormality

Minimal set of investigations for UTI

1. Urine dipstick
2. MSU—specimen collection may involve a clean catch (in boys), collection bag (most common but not ideal),

catheterization (invasive), and suprapubic aspiration. Samples must undergo standard microscopy and culture

3. USS—the initial radiological investigation of choice for examination of entire renal tract
4. MCUG—indicated routinely in all patients under the age of 2 years, but also in >2-year-olds if history of febrile illness, recurrent UTI, or renal scarring
5. Static (DMSA) renal scintigraphy—indications the same as MCUG

Additional investigations
1. KUB—if renal calculi suspected
2. IVU—rarely used, but useful in stone disease and to demonstrate renal tract anatomy
3. Cystoscopy—not used routinely, but may be indicated for the diagnosis of suspected urethral valves, ureteroceles, bladder, or urethral diverticulum

---

(c) POSTERIOR URETHRAL VALVES (PUV)

Overview
- Comprise membranous mucosal folds which obstruct urine flow during micturition
- Most common obstructive lesion of the urethra in children
- Incidence of 1 in 4,000–8,000
- Only occur in males
- >80% are detected pre-natally—fetal USS detects a persistently distended bladder and bilateral upper tract obstruction
- Found at the level of the distal prostatic urethra
- Typically, the membrane arises from the veru montanum and extends anteriorly through the area of the external urethral sphincter to attach to the anterior urethral wall
- PUV are classified into 3 types:
  - Type I (95%)—opening positioned near the veru montanum
  - Type II—not obstructive and doubts exist as to its existence
  - Type III (5%)—incomplete dissolution of the urogenital membrane

Post-natally, the infant or child may present with—

- Obstructive LUTS—poor flow, prolonged voiding, frequency
- Distended bladder
- UTI

- Renal failure—growth retardation, failure to thrive
- Generally unwell—irritable, listless

Minimal set of investigations for PUV
1. MSSU—often confirms infection
2. Blood tests—may demonstrate an elevated serum creatinine and urea
3. USS—primary radiological investigation. Findings include a distended, thickened, bladder; upper tract dilatation; dilated posterior urethra; perinephric urinoma
4. MCUG—best method of diagnosing and defining the anatomy of PUV. Will also assess the presence of ureteric reflux (presence in up to 60% of cases)

Additional investigations
1. Renal function assessment—using radionuclide isotopic GFR or creatinine clearance if renal failure suspected
2. Cystoscopy—direct visual identification establishes the diagnosis and may also permit endoscopic valve ablation

---

(d) UNDESCENDED TESTIS (UDT)

Overview
- Incidence at birth is between 3.4% and 5.8% at birth
- Incidence drops to 0.8% by the age of 1 year
- Well-recognized manifestation of over 50 congenital syndromes
- Approximately 25% of cases are bilateral
- UDT is broadly classified into—
  - Palpable (80%)
  - Non-palpable (20%)
    - Intra-abdominal (10%)
    - Atrophic (6%)
    - Absent (4%)

The diagnosis is usually made on clinical examination at birth, but all patients must be followed up with serial examination up to the age of 2 years. Spontaneous descent will occur in over 70% within the first year of life (mainly within the first 6 months). A distinction must be made between UDT and retractile testis, which is traditionally regarded as a variant of normal. Surgical intervention between 12 and 18 months is indicated if UDT persists due to risks of subfertility and malignant change.

Investigations for UDT

If the cryptorchidism is unilateral (with a normal contralateral testis) or bilateral, further tests may be useful but are not essential.

If unilateral UDT

1. Radiography—USS or MRI scan may help locate the absent testis. The accuracy of USS can be as low as 0–50% for intra-abdominal testis, but is considerably better for MRI scan (90%)
2. Laparoscopy—is the procedure of choice if intra-abdominal retention of testis is suspected and is a useful diagnostic and therapeutic procedure

If bilateral UDT

1. Endocrine tests
   —abnormally elevated serum FSH and LH level with absent testosterone is consistent with anorchia
   —serum FSH, LH and testosterone may be slightly low in true bilateral UDT
   —serum FSH, LH, and testosterone grossly decreased in primary hypopituitarism
   —if bilateral UDT persists after 3 months of age, a human chorionic gonadotrophin (HCG) stimulation test should be performed. This includes measurement of baseline serum testosterone, followed by 4 days of HCG (2,000 units), and then a repeat testosterone estimation. At least a ten-fold increase in testosterone suggests functioning testis, while no significant increase is diagnostic of anorchia
2. Laparoscopy—if intra-abdominal testes suspected, laparoscopic exploration is essential

---

(e) URINARY INCONTINENCE

Overview

- Day- or nighttime urinary incontinence is common in children
- By the age of 7 years, 6% of girls and 3.8% of boys continue to have problems with daytime incontinence
- Can be classified as either nocturnal or diurnal; functional or organic
- An organic etiology is uncommon but must be excluded
- Primary nocturnal enuresis is rarely due to an organic factor

- Continuous leakage almost always has an organic etiology
- Children who were once dry but subsequently developed incontinence virtually never demonstrate an anatomical abnormality
- A detailed history and physical examination are the most important factors in reaching a satisfactory diagnosis
- Some of the causes of incontinence (with pattern of wetting) include—
  - Organic
    - UTI (incontinence intermittent)
    - Neurogenic bladder (intermittent or continuous)
    - Bladder outflow obstruction (intermittent)
    - Anatomical, e.g., bladder extrophy, ectopic ureter (intermittent or continuous)
  - Functional (almost always intermittent)
    - Dysfunctional voiding
    - Urge syndrome
    - Primary nocturnal enuresis
    - Lazy bladder
    - Hinman's syndrome
    - Diurnal enuresis

Minimal set of investigations for pediatric incontinence
1. MSU—to exclude infection
2. USS—allows rapid assessment of entire urinary tract

Additional investigations
These are rarely required for isolated symptoms of incontinence because the baseline investigations are adequate to reassure both the physician and patient/parents in most cases. These tests are only suitable for older children, who are able to comply with simple instructions. Indications for advanced testing include—

- Suspected neurogenic bladder
- Continued troublesome symptoms without a satisfactory diagnosis
- Stress incontinence
- Suspected anatomical abnormality of the lower urinary tract

1. Video-urodynamics
2. Frequency voiding chart—useful for objective assessment and biofeedback, but often not practical

Chapter 12
Andrology

(a) ERECTILE DYSFUNCTION (ED)

Overview
- Affects at least half of all men over the age of 40 years to some degree
- Prevalence of moderate to severe ED increases with age (see Table 12.1)
- Erectile function is a complex mechanism
- ED is a multi-factorial phenomenon—factors are rarely present in isolation but commonly occur in a synergistic combination
- Causative factors can be broadly classified as—
  - Psychogenic—due to a variety of stressful psychological and lifestyle problems
  - Organic
    a. *Vascular*—most common cause. Risk factors include hypertension, diabetes mellitus, atherosclerosis, hyperlipidemia, obesity, pelvic injury, and smoking
    b. *Neurogenic*—causes include diabetes mellitus, alcoholism, multiple sclerosis, stroke, depression, Parkinson's disease, spinal cord injury, brain trauma
    c. *Endocrine*—androgen deficiency and hyperprolactinemia
    d. *Drug-induced*—a large proportion of therapeutic and recreational drugs may cause ED, especially cardiac, hormonal, and psychotropic medications
    e. *Structural*—Peyronie's disease, penile fracture, congenital penile abnormalities
    f. *Iatrogenic*—pelvic surgery or radiotherapy, TURP, medications
    g. *Systemic disease*—renal failure, liver cirrhosis, chronic debilitation, etc.

TABLE 12.1. Prevalence of ED with increasing age

Age (ys)	Approximate prevalence (%)
40–49	10
50–59	20
60–69	40
>70	>60

Investigations
- Most men with ED do not require extensive investigations
- Nevertheless, baseline assessment is mandatory in order to define the extent and potential risk factors in such patients

Minimal set of investigations for ED
- Full physical examination
  - Abdomen, external genitalia, and rectal
  - Global endocrine function—body habitus, hair distribution
  - Femoral and lower limb arterial pulses
  - Perineal and lower neurology

- Assessment using standardised questionnaires
  - Psychosexual and medical
  - Standardized questionnaire (e.g., International index of erectile function) will allow objective analysis of disease severity

- Appropriate laboratory tests
  - Urine dipstick—to detect glucosuria or hematuria
  - MSSU—to exclude infection
  - Full blood count
  - Fasting blood glucose—diabetes mellitus
  - Fasting lipid profile—hyperlipidemia
  - Morning serum testosterone—hypogonadism
  - Prolactin—hyperprolactinemia

Additional investigations
Although the majority of patients need no further assessment other than a baseline evaluation, indications for advanced tests include—

- Patient request
- Medicolegal cases

- Absence of any obvious disorder (psychogenic or organic)
- Suspicion of endocrine disorder (e.g., hypogonadism, hyperprolactinemia)
- If surgical intervention is being considered in a patient with suspected vascular insufficiency
- In patients with structural/congenital penile deformities
- Patients with complex psychiatric or psychological illness

Types of advanced tests are summarized in Table 12.2.

(b) PEYRONIE'S DISEASE

- Benign penile condition
- Prevalence—0.4% to 1% in middle-aged men
- Characterized by abnormal fibrosis within the tunica albuginea
- Classically consists of two phases (early/inflammatory and late/stable)
- May present with—
  - Pain of erection
  - Penile angulation or deviation when rigid
  - Palpable penile plaques
  - Penile shortening
  - ED
- Formal investigations usually not required
- An accurate record must be made of the number, size, location, and consistency of penile plaques
- Indications for formal assessment include—
  - Presence of complex deformities
  - If surgery is being considered
  - Monitoring of medical therapy
  - Persistence of diagnostic doubt
  - As part of a research protocol

Advanced investigations for Peyronie's disease are summarized in Table 12.3.

(c) SUB-FERTILITY

- Inability to conceive after 1 year of unprotected intercourse
- Male factors solely responsible for 20% of cases and play a contributory role in another 30%
- Both partners should be investigated simultaneously, since female factors such as age, previous pregnancies, and medical

TABLE 12.2. Advanced tests for ED

Tests	Comments
Endocrine	Serum FSH and LH if testosterone low Thyroid function tests
Nocturnal penile tumescence and rigidity	Tumescence and rigidity can be measured at the base and tip of penis using the Rigiscan Can help differentiate between psychogenic and organic ED Testing for at least 2 days Normal—at least two nocturnal erections; erections with at least 60% rigidity at penile tip, lasting >10 min
Intracavernous injection	Assessment of vascular sufficiency (arterial and venous) Cavernous injection of 10 µg of alprostadil or prostaglandin Normal—rigid erection within 10 min of injection and lasting for >30 min
Penile duplex ultrasound	Assessment of vascular sufficiency (arterial and venous) Cavernous injection of 10 µg of alprostadil or prostaglandin Normal • Peak systolic velocity (PSV) >30 cm/s • Resistive index >0.8 Abnormal • PSV <25 cm/s PSV >30 cm/s and the end diastolic velocity >3 cm/s is suggestive of venous leakage
Arteriography	Penile arteriography (for anatomical information) should only be considered if vascular reconstructive surgery is planned
Dynamic infusion cavernosometry and cavernosography	If venous leakage is suspected to be the cause of ED
Psychiatric assessment	Consider if significant psychiatric disorder

history will certainly have a direct effect on the chances of conception

The following table describes the etiological factors responsible for male infertility (Table 12.4).

TABLE 12.3. Further investigations for Peyronie's disease

Test	Comments
Stretched penile length	Corresponds reasonably well to erect penile length
Measurement of penile deviation	Following an induced erection (using intracavernosal injection), the angle of deviation can be measured with a goniometer
Polaroid photographs	Useful if patient declines artificial erection, but prone to inaccuracies
Plain radiography	Help delineate calcified plaque in the penis
Ultrasound	Rarely used as findings do not correlate with clinical situation. Can assess plaque and any other corporal fibrosis
Dupplex ultrasound	Useful in evaluation of associated ED since arterio-venous insufficiency is found in 8–86% of patients
Penile scintigraphy	Can distinguish between early and late phase of disease. 370 MBq of ^{99m}Tc-human IgG injected. Tracer accumulates in areas of active inflammatory response
MRI	Will accurately detect plaque but rarely clinically indicated

TABLE 12.4. Etiology of male infertility

Etiological cause	Frequency (%)
Idiopathic abnormal semen (no demonstrable cause)	75.1
Varicocele	12.3
Urogenital infection	6.6
Immunological factors	3.1
Acquired factors	2.6
Congenital anomalies	2.1
Sexual factors	1.7
Endocrine disturbances	0.6
Other abnormalities	3.0

TABLE 12.5. Additional tests for investigation of male infertility

Test	Indications	Comments
Computer-assisted semen analysis	Indicated if significant discrepancy between serial manual SA	Aims to improve subjective variations Most useful for assessing sperm motility
Endocrine evaluation (testosterone, FSH, LH, Prolactin)	If sperm count <10 million/mL Impaired sexual function (e.g., impotence) Other findings suggesting a specific endocrine disorder	Endocrine problem is very uncommon if semen analysis normal
Post-ejaculate urinalysis for sperm	If ejaculate volumes <1 ml	Microscopic examination of urine for sperm helps exclude retrograde ejaculation
Semen leukocyte analysis	If SA shows increased number of WBC	Immunocytology will help differentiate WBC from immature sperm Pyospermia >1 million WBC/mL Suggests infection or inflammation
Post-coital test	If hyperviscous sperm Infertile despite normal SA Abnormal penile anatomy (e.g., hypospadias)	Microscopic examination of cervical mucous shortly after intercourse Assessment of interaction between sperm and female partner cervical mucus

TABLE 12.5. *Continued*

Test	Indications	Comments
Anti-sperm antibodies	If isolated asthenospermia (poor motility) If sperm agglutination Abnormal post-coital test Unexplained infertility	Normal >10 progressive sperm/hpf The finding of antibodies on the spermatozoon surface is more significant than antibodies in serum
Sperm viability test	If poor sperm motility	Hypoosmotic swelling test Will identify non-motile but viable sperm for assisted fertilization techniques
Sperm penetration assay	Unexplained infertility, if couple considering assisted reproduction (AR)	Sperm penetration analysis using hamster eggs Normal >10% of eggs penetrated and >5 penetrations per egg Good penetration correlated with improved success with AR
Radiological **Vasography**	If obstruction is suspected	Is not an isolated procedure and may be performed at the time of surgery
Scrotal USS (7.5–10 mHz frequency)	Abnormal physical scrotal examination	May identify relevant scrotal pathologies including varicocele, cysts, absent vas and testicular masses

TABLE 12.5. *Continued*

Test	Indications	Comments
TRUSS	To exclude ejaculatory duct obstruction if azoospermia or oligospermia, low ejaculate volumes and palpable vas	Normal findings include seminal vesicle diameter of <1.5 cm and non-dilated ejaculatory ducts
CT/MRI	Rarely indicated but useful if solitary right-sided varicocele (to exclude retroperitoneal pathology)	
Genetic testing	If non-obstructive azoospermia or severe oligospermia (<5 million sperm/mL). If genetic abnormality is suspected. Prior to performing intracytoplasmic sperm injection (ICSI)	The most common genetic abnormalities include— • Cystic fibrosis gene mutations (associated with congenital bilateral absence of the vas deferens) • Klinefelter's syndrome (karyotype abnormalities) • Y-chromosome deletions
Testicular biopsy	To differentiate between obstructive and non-obstructive azoospermia, if no obvious other abnormality. As part of a therapeutic process if ICSI is being considered	Biopsy may be performed using— • Open technique • Percutaneously • Testicular sperm extraction (TESE) • Microscopic epididymal sperm extraction (MESE)

Indications for fertility assessment
- Infertile patient
- Assessment may be commenced prior to the completion of 1 year as defined by the infertility criteria for certain situations:

  - If known existing male fertility risk factor (e.g., previous bilateral cryptorchidism)
  - If the couple are anxious to establish male fertility potential, especially if female partner age is increased

Minimal set of investigations
- Full history and physical examination (including pelvic examination)
- MSSU—(exclude infection, hematuria, etc)
- Semen analysis (SA) × 2—since infertility is practically defined as an abnormal semen analysis, this remains the cornerstone of evaluation and forms the basis of important decisions concerning appropriate further investigations. (See Chapter 6h—Semen analysis)

Additional investigations
- Not routinely indicated—justified if results are likely to change patient management
- Indicated if semen analysis shows an obvious abnormality requiring further amplification
- Such investigations are intrusive, time-consuming, and expensive

A brief summary of other adjunctive tests is given in the Table 12.5.

Index